Hand-Held and Automated BREAST ULTRASOUND

Institute of Cancer Research Library

Lawrence W. Bassett, MD
Associate Professor of Radiological Sciences
UCLA School of Medicine
Los Angeles, California

—

Richard H. Gold, MD
Professor of Radiological Sciences
UCLA School of Medicine
Los Angeles, California

—

Carolyn Kimme-Smith, PhD
Adjunct Assistant Professor of Radiological Sciences
UCLA School of Medicine
Los Angeles, California

Hand-Held and Automated
BREAST ULTRASOUND

Lawrence W. Bassett, MD
Richard H. Gold, MD
Carolyn Kimme-Smith, PhD

SLACK 6900 Grove Road • Thorofare, New Jersey 08086

Copyright© 1986 by SLACK Incorporated

All rights reserved. No part of this book may be reproduced, stored in a retrieval system or transmitted in any form or by any means, electronic, mechanical, photocopying, recorded or otherwise, without written permission from the publisher, except for brief quotations embodied in critical articles and reviews.

Printed in the United States of America

Library of Congress Catalog Card Number: 85-61595

ISBN: 0-943432-53-7

Published by: Slack Incorporated
            6900 Grove Road
            Thorofare, NJ 08086

Last digit is print number: 8   7   6   5   4   3   2   1

CONTENTS

Foreword *vii*

Preface *ix*

1. Introduction *1*
   Historical perspectives *3*
   Evaluation of breast masses *3*
   Breast cancer detection/diagnosis *4*
   Additional clinical indications *5*
   Hand-held real-time versus automated scanning *5*
   Cost-effectiveness *6*
   Future developments *7*

2. Physics *11*
   Introduction *13*
   How the image is formed *13*
   Ultrasound imaging compared to x-ray imaging *14*
   Transducers *16*
   Attenuation *23*
   Time gain compensation and power *24*
   Reflection and refraction *27*

3. Instrumentation and Technique *33*
   Introduction *35*
   Signal processing *35*
   Hand-held real-time instrumentation *40*
   Automated instruments *49*
   Quality control and calibration *57*

4. The Normal Breast *61*
   Introduction *63*
   Anatomy *63*
   Ultrasound of the normal breast *63*
   The pregnant breast *78*

5. Benign Disorders *81*

Introduction *83*
Cysts *83*
Fibroadenoma *90*
Cystosarcoma phylloides *92*
Intraductal papilloma *95*
Lipoma *95*
Abscess *98*
Galactocele *99*
Sebaceous cyst *99*
Hematoma *99*
Other biopsy changes *99*
Breast augmentation mammoplasty *104*

6. Malignant Lesions *107*

Introduction *109*
Ultrasound features of breast carcinomas *109*
Histologic-sonographic correlation of breast carcinomas *117*
Metastatic cancer to the breast *125*
Sarcomas *126*

7. Pitfalls and How To Avoid Them *129*

Introduction *131*
Pitfalls in interpreting the examination *131*
Pitfalls in performing the examination *135*

8. Quiz Cases *143*

Appendix. Physics and Instrumentation Terms Defined *187*

Index *201*

FOREWORD

This textbook on the use of breast ultrasound imaging is especially important, coming as it does at a time when clinicians are searching for more accurate methods of diagnosing breast disease. The authors have already documented in numerous publications their extensive experience in x-ray mammography. Now to aid clinicians who are faced with the problems of equivocal x-ray mammograms or abnormal radiographic findings that are not clinically apparent, they have taken the diagnosis of breast disease a step further by sharing their personal experience in the use of ultrasound imaging as an adjunct to x-ray mammography. The subject is covered from the pioneering use of A-mode analysis of breast masses to the present day sophistication of high-resolution hand-held real-time units and high frequency units dedicated to the automated examination of the entire breast.

A knowledge of the physics of the interaction of ultrasound in breast tissue is required to interpret normal and abnormal ultrasound images and to permit an objective evaluation of ultrasound equipment and techniques. It is not surprising, therefore, that x-ray mammographers who have failed to acquire such knowledge usually have been disinterested in ultrasound imaging, preferring to relegate it to their colleagues who specialize in general ultrasonography. This textbook supplies among other things sufficient information regarding physics and instrumentation to enable the x-ray mammographer to become an ultrasound mammographer as well. To allow familiarization with normal ultrasound patterns, the reader will also find images of normal breasts at different ages. Alterations from normal patterns are correlated with benign or malignant disease, and numerous sonographic examples of varying pathologic abnormalities are described and illustrated.

Many years were required for dedicated investigators to develop the use of x-ray mammography. Finally, with the development of appropriate pathologic correlation and careful biostatistical guidelines, x-ray mammography entered the radiological armamentarium and became part of the curriculum of radiological and x-ray technological training programs throughout the country. And now with the development of multimodality breast imaging centers, x-ray mammographers have begun to show interest in understanding the interactions of sound and breast tissue. Since many private radiological offices, clinics and hospitals already have general purpose equipment for abdominal and obstetrical ultrasound, it is certain that with the increasing availability of higher frequency transducers, preferably with water delay mechanisms, increasing attention will be devoted to breast ultrasonography.

For the radiologists involved in the evaluation of breast disease, the use of ultrasound imaging should increase diagnostic accuracy and decrease the number of breast biopsies. The addition of sonographic information is most valuable in the differentiation of cysts and solid masses. Small fluid-filled cysts can be reliably diagnosed. Although the same high level of diagnostic accuracy is not possible in the differentiation of benign and malignant solid masses, if further refinements in diagnosis are to be made an understanding of current diagnostic criteria for solid lesions is essential. It is even conceivable that background echo patterns may in the future serve as tissue signatures to identify a breast that is likely or unlikely to harbor or develop a cancer.

As this book clearly indicates, breast ultrasound is no longer in its infant state, but is rather a diagnostic modality that has truly come into its own.

Catherine Cole-Beuglet, MD, FRCP(C)
Professor of Radiology
University of California, Irvine

PREFACE

As ultrasound has gradually become an accepted adjunct to x-ray mammography, many x-ray mammographers have expressed frustration with the uneven quality and variability of the images produced by a wide range of ultrasound instruments. The variations in breast parenchyma that may be encountered in the normal population are represented by a broad spectrum of ultrasound images. Published sonograms of proven pathology often show only subtle alterations from these normal images. Since the ultrasound image results from the reflections of sound waves from the surface and from within the breast rather than from its transmission or absorption of radiation, and since the ultrasound image delineates a slice rather than a single projection of the entire breast, it is not surprising that ultrasound complements rather than reproduces x-ray mammographic findings.

Ultrasound images may be misdiagnosed because of inappropriate scanning techniques or because of unfamiliarity with ultrasonic diagnostic signs and the scanning methods that record them. Ultrasonic instruments have proliferated as rapidly as the microprocessor chips they utilize, resulting in an array of options and special purpose instruments that tend to lead to further diagnostic confusion.

With these problems in mind, we have divided this book into eight chapters: Introduction, Physics, Instrumentation and Technique, The Normal Breast, Benign Disorders, Malignant Lesions, Pitfalls and How To Avoid Them, and Quiz Cases. We have included a glossary of common terms used in ultrasound physics and instrumentation.

A working knowledge of physics, instrumentation and technique is essential to a full understanding of ultrasound mammography, and will hopefully prevent many of the pitfalls described in Chapter 7. Considerable space has been devoted to the real-time hand-held technique, since it is the one most widely used to evaluate palpable breast masses. Nevertheless, numerous whole-breast automated images are illustrated, and the machines that produced them are fully described and compared.

We hope that this book will prove a useful guide to physicians who perform and interpret breast sonograms, to their technologists, and most of all, to those physicians and technologists who have yet to gain experience in ultrasound technique and interpretation, and evaluation of breast imaging equipment.

ACKNOWLEDGMENTS

We thank Delma Westbrook, CRT, our dedicated ultrasound mammography technologist. In addition to performing ultrasound examinations of excellent quality, she spent many hours collecting cases to illustrate this book.

We are grateful to the following investigators for the cases they contributed: Drs. Catherine Cole-Beuglet, Elizabeth Kelly-Fry, Wende W. Logan, Marjorie B. McSweeney, Louise O'Shaugnessy, Edward E. Sickles, and Joel Sokoloff.

In addition, we give credit to our ultrasound associates—Drs. William King III and Dennis A. Sarti who performed many of the examinations used in this textbook.

Finally, we are grateful to our secretary, Mary Frazier, for her assistance and dedication to the completion of this book.

CHAPTER 1

Introduction

HISTORICAL PERSPECTIVES

The usefulness of ultrasound for breast diagnosis was discovered over 30 years ago by Wild and Reid[1] and Howry, et al,[2] who demonstrated its potential for differentiating cystic from solid breast masses by A-mode technique. Later, Kratchowil and Kaiser[3] found contact scanning with conventional B-mode equipment useful in the evaluation of palpable masses. Subsequently, DeLand,[4] Baum,[5] Jellins, Kossoff et al,[6] Kobayashi,[7] and Kelly-Fry[8] developed automated water-path breast ultrasound scanners for examination of the whole breast.

EVALUATION OF BREAST MASSES

The primary indication for breast ultrasound is the evaluation of masses detected on physical examination or mammography. In this endeavor, accuracy rates of 96% to 100% have been reported in differentiating cysts from solid masses.[9-11] Pragmatists would argue that a needle aspiraton of cyst fluid is faster, less expensive, and therapeutic as well as diagnostic. However, one would hesitate to aspirate all cysts that are diagnosed unequivocally by ultrasound; multiple cysts would require numerous aspirations that could be both uncomfortable and traumatic for the patient. The greatest usefulness of sonography is when cyst-solid differentiation is required for a mammographically-detected nonpalpable, noncalcified mass of indeterminate origin for which aspiration is impractical.

Breast sonography can often differentiate benign from malignant solid masses, but its sensitivity and specificity in this regard is much lower than for cyst-solid differentiation. The sonographic features used to distinguish benign and malignant masses are not sufficiently reliable to defer biopsy of a solid mass. Indeed, all solid masses must be considered potentially malignant.

BREAST CANCER DETECTION/ DIAGNOSIS

Automated breast sonography has been advocated as a screening device for breast cancer, with reported detection rates approaching those of x-ray mammography.[12-15] However, in many of these studies x-ray mammograms were performed only when there was a palpable or sonographic abnormality. In other studies, clinical data was available for interpretation of sonomammograms but not for interpretation of x-ray mammograms. In some studies, the ability of sonography to differentiate solid from cystic masses was compared with the ability of mammography to specifically indicate malignancy. Thus, the accuracy of ultrasound mammography relative to x-ray mammography has been overestimated in the literature.

More recently, investigators have reported a significant number of nonpalpable cancers detected by x-ray mammography but missed by ultrasound mammography.[13,16] These studies have pointed out the limitations of ultrasound in the detection of breast cancer: 1) poor results in fatty breasts; 2) inability of ultrasound to depict microcalcifications, often the earliest x-ray sign of breast cancer; 3) inconsistent identification of solid lesions under 1cm in diameter; and 4) unreliable ultrasound criteria for distinction of benign and malignant solid masses. When compared with x-ray mammography for breast cancer screening, automated breast ultrasound is also limited by relatively long technologist scanning time, physician reviewing time, and dedicated equipment costs. Because of these limitations, ultrasound is currently not considered useful as a primary screening modality for breast cancer detection.

Ultrasonography is most accurate in breasts that are dense in mammograms and difficult to evaluate by either film-screen or xeromammography. The combined use of x-ray and ultrasound mammography has been shown to improve the detection rate for breast cancer.[17] Therefore, breast ultrasound should be considered an adjunct to but not a substitute for mammography and physical examination in the detection and diagnosis of breast cancer.[18]

ADDITIONAL CLINICAL INDICATIONS

Ultrasound is helpful in the evaluation of uniformly dense breasts in which noncalcified cancers may be undetected by x-ray mammography. Breast ultrasound has been proposed as the initial screening procedure for women under age 35 in whom the breasts tend to be dense and the false-negative rate for x-ray mammography is high.[19] Because it has not been associated with harmful effects, sonography can be used frequently in the evaluation of dense nodular fibrocystic breasts, which are often ill-suited to physical examination and mammography.

Ultrasound is useful for the evaluation of patients with cystic disease in whom the large number and varying size of the cysts preclude needle aspiration. In these patients, sonography can be used for evaluation of the response to therapy.[20]

Ultrasound is helpful in the evaluation of patients with breast augmentation prostheses, in whom the usefulness of x-ray mammography and physical examination is limited.[21]

Ultrasound-guided aspiration biopsy of nonpalpable lesions has been shown to be effective, and the method has also been advocated for prebiopsy needle localization of nonpalpable masses.[22]

HAND-HELD REAL-TIME VERSUS AUTOMATED SCANNING

Hand-held real-time units are most useful when attention can be directed to a specific area of the breast. For the evaluation of palpable masses, many hand-held real-time units having a transducer frequency at or above 5MHz can identify simple cysts, thereby averting unnecessary biopsies.

Hand-held units are also applicable to patients with palpable masses and indeterminate findings on x-ray mammography.[23] Advantages over automated units include improved resolution due to the higher frequency of the transducer, ability to vary the amount of compression to assess tissue compliance and mass fixation, and usefulness in guiding needle aspiration biopsies. A disadvantage is poor penetration, lack of anatomical labeling, and decreased resolution near the transducer. The latter problem can be solved by attaching a water-path step-off device to the transducer.

Automated water-path instruments designed specifically for whole-breast examination make it possible to systemically examine the breast in its entirety. This type of equipment is required when breast ultrasound is used to search for nonpalpable lesions.[24] Current automated units use single or multiple transducers with frequencies of 3.9 to 4.5MHz. These units achieve a resolution on the order of 2mm. To identify small lesions it is necessary to scan at close intervals, which results in multiple sequential images of separate slices of the breast. It is also desirable to be able to compare images of both breasts at similar planes. This is usually accomplished by dual-videotape or videodisc playback of the examination.

COST-EFFECTIVENESS

Ultrasound examinations can be performed immediately following the mammographic examination. In our clinical setting, the radiologist determines the need for an ultrasound evaluation of a palpable or mammographic mass, and the examination is performed at the initial visit. This mechanism has been acceptable to referring physicians and patients. Since the ultrasound evaluation frequently results in a biopsy that is more timely if not entirely deferred, it is considered to be cost-effective. Some referring physicians request the radiologist to proceed without formal consultation to ultrasound-guided aspiration of a mammographically or ultrasonically detected nonpalpable cyst.

Due to the high cost of dedicated automated breast units and the additional time required for whole breast evaluation, the cost per examination usually equals or exceeds that of x-ray mammography. Although automated breast sonography sometimes provides clinically relevant information when used as an adjunct to physical examination and x-ray mammography, and occasionally is the only method to detect a carcinoma in a dense breast, the high cost of the examination precludes its routine use. Therefore, specific clinical situations need to be defined for which the addition of automated ultrasound mammography may be cost-effective. The most promising application appears to be the evaluation of multiple palpable masses in radiographically dense breasts. We customarily perform automated breast ultrasound examinations in cases where the x-ray mammograms are significantly compromised by dense parenchymal tissue.

FUTURE DEVELOPMENTS

Many independent investigators are currently evaluating the clinical applications of breast ultrasound. This unfortunately has led to considerable variability in protocols, instrumentation, image quality, and diagnostic accuracy. To date, most subjects have been symptomatic, and data for an entirely asymptomatic population has yet to be acquired. A multi-institutional study of image interpretation with properly controlled technical and biostatistical procedures is needed.

Ultrasonic computerized axial tomography (UCAT) is now under development in an attempt to provide more quantitative data relative to the production of ultrasound images of the breast.[25,26] Related techniques such as backscatter and transmission computerized sonography, combining data of the velocity and relative attenuation of sound through the breast, are currently under investigation. Although UCAT appears promising, problems include image distortion produced by nonuniform refractive indices and the influence of surrounding tissues upon sound velocity through lesions. Like x-ray mammography, UCAT is less effective for cancer detection in the dense breast.

Doppler systems are being used on an experimental basis to study the vascular physiology of the breast and breast tumors. Preliminary work has shown that Doppler signals from carcinoma differ from those obtained from normal breast tissue.[27]

Tissue characterization, based on investigations of the interactions of sonic waves with breast tissues of differing types and combinations, continues to be investigated. The effect of collagen, mucin, mucopolysaccharides and other biologic substances on image formation and, specifically, on the sonographic appearance of cancer must be further defined.[28] These breast studies will require correlation with x-ray mammography, specimen radiography, and pathology.[29]

Efforts continue toward improving the resolution of dedicated breast ultrasound scanners. Pulse echo scanners may benefit from higher frequency transducers, provided they maintain penetration sufficient to image the entire breast. Some manufacturers are investigating the use of polyvinyl layered transducers for both automated and real-time breast scanners.

Improved resolution can also be achieved by image processing methods that are now available through the development of high speed, inexpensive, special purpose microprocessors. An annular array transducer is being studied for breast echography[30]; this configuration improves both transverse and slice thickness resolution without affecting penetration. Microprocessors can also be used to correct for the smearing of signals received from echoes located deep within the breast. Methods exist for correcting distortions of both the width dimension of the echoes received and the length of the echo smeared by its travel through the breast.[31,32]

Other image processing methods can reduce the graininess characteristic of ultrasound images. These patterns of uneven texture are independent of the tissues; they vary from frame to frame even when the transducer moves repeatedly over the same section of the breast. Methods to reduce ultrasonic speckle[33] are being incorporated into many of the newest ultrasonic scanners.

References

1. Wild JJ, Reid JM: Further pilot echographic studies on the histologic structure of the living intact human breast. Am J Pathol 28:839-854, 1952.
2. Howry DM, Stott DA, Bliss WR: The ultrasonic visualization of carcinoma of the breast and other soft tissue structures. Cancer 7:354-358, 1954.
3. Kratchowil A, Kaiser P: Die Darstellung der Erkrankungen der weiblichen Brust im Ultraschallschnittbildverfahren, In Bock J, Ossoining K (eds): Ultrasono Graphia Medica, Vol III. Verlag der Weiner Medizinischen Akademie, Vienna, 1969, pp 119-126.
4. Deland FH: A modified technique of ultrasonography for the detection and differential diagnosis of breast lesions. AJR 105:446-452, 1969.
5. Baum G: A comparison of the performance of commercial ultrasound breast scanners versus a laboratory instrument. JCU 10:159-166, 1982.
6. Jellins J, Kossoff G, Buddee FW, et al: Ultrasonic visualization of the breast. Med J Aust 1:305-307, 1971.
7. Kobayashi T: Ultrasonic diagnosis of breast cancer. Ultrasound Med Biol 1:383-391, 1975.
8. Kelly-Fry E: Breast Imaging, In Sabbagha RE (ed): Ultrasound Applied to Obstetrics and Gynecology. Harper & Row, New York, 1980, pp 327-350.
9. Rosner D, Weiss L, Norman M: Ultrasonography in the diagnosis of breast disease. J Surg Oncology 14:83-96, 1980.
10. Sickles EA, Filly RA, Callen PW: Benign breast lesions: ultrasound detection and diagnosis. Radiology 151:467-470, 1984.
11. Fleischner AC, Muhletaler CA, Reynolds, VH, et al: Palpable breast masses: Evaluation by high frequency, hand-held real-time sonography and xeromammography. Radiology 148:813-817, 1983.
12. Pluygers E, Rombaut M: Ultrasonic diagnosis of breast diseases. Tumor Diagnostik 4:187-194, 1980.
13. Kobayashi T, Takatani O, Hattori N, et al: Differential diagnosis of breast tumors: The sensitivity graded method of ultrasonography and clinical evaluation of its diagnostic accuracy. Cancer 33:940-951, 1974.
14. Devere C: Current status of ultrasonic breast scanning. Applied Radiology 145-149, 1980.
15. Cole-Beuglet C, Goldberg BB, Kurtz AB, et al: Ultrasound mammography. Radiology 139:693-698, 1981.
16. Sickles EA, Filly FA, Callen PW: Breast cancer detection with ultrasonography and mammography: Comparison using state-of-the-art equipment. AJR 140:843-845, 1983.

17. Teixidor HS, Kazam E: Combined mammographic-sonographic evaluation of breast masses. AJR 128:409-417, 1977.

18. Gold RH, Sickles EA, Bassett LW, et al: Diagnostic imaging of the breast. Investigative Radiology 19 (Suppl):S43-S59,1984.

19. Harper AP, Kelly-Fry E, Noe S: Ultrasound breast imaging—the method of choice for examining the young patient. Ultrasound in Medicine and Biology 7:231-237, 1981.

20. Sickles EA, Filly RA, Callen PW: Breast ultrasonography, In Feig SA, McLelland R (eds): Breast Carcinoma: Current Diagnosis and Treatment. Masson, New York, 1983.

21. Cole-Beuglet C, Schwartz G, Kurtz AB: Ultrasound mammography for the augmented breast. Radiology 146:737-742, 1983.

22. Kopans DB, Meyer JE, Lindfors KL, et al: Breast sonography to guide cyst aspiration and wire localization of occult solid lesions. AJR 143:489, 1984.

23. Rubin E, Miller VE, Berland LL, et al: Hand-held real-time breast sonography. AJR 144:623-627, 1985.

24. McSweeney MB, Murphy CH: Whole-breast sonography. Radiol Clin North Am 23:157-167, 1985.

25. Greenleaf JF, Bahn RC: Clinical imaging with transmissive ultrasonic computerized tomography. IEEE Transactions on Biomedical Engineering 28:177-185, 1981.

26. Carson PL, Meyer CR, Scherzinger AL, et al: Breast imaging in coronal planes with simultaneous pulse echo and transmission ultrasound. Science 214:1141-1143, 1981.

27. Bamber JC: Ultrasonic tissue characteristics in cancer diagnosis and management. RNM Images 12-19, 1983.

28. Cole-Beuglet C, Soriano RZ, Kurtz AB, et al: Ultrasound analysis of 104 primary breast carcinomas classified according to histopathologic type. Radiology 147:191-196, 1983.

29. Teubner J, Muller A, van Kaick G: Echomorophologie der Brustdruse. Vergleichende sonographische, radiologische, anatomische und histologische. Untersuchungen von Mamapraparaten. Radiologe 23:97-107, 1983.

30. Arditi M, Taylor WB, Taster FS, et al: An annular array system for high resolution breast echography. Ultrasonic Imaging 4:1-31, 1982.

31. Robinson DE, Wing M: Lateral deconvolution of ultrasonic beams. Ultrasonic Imaging 6:1-12, 1984.

32. Demoment G, Raynaud R, Herment A: Range resolution improvement by a fast deconvolution method. Ultrasonic Imaging 6:435-451, 1984.

33. Sommer FG, Sue JY: Image processing to reduce ultrasonic speckle. J Ultrasound Med 413-416, 1983.

CHAPTER 2

Physics

INTRODUCTION

In order to successfully interpret breast ultrasound examinations it is essential to understand the underlying physical principles of reflection, scattering, and absorption of sound waves by the breast tissues. Ultrasound is the only imaging modality that employs energy reflection, rather than energy transmission. In addition, it is the only imaging examination in which the energy source is also the receiver. Unlike an x-ray mammogram, the sonogram is dependent on the elasticity as well as the density of the breast tissues.

This chapter explains the physical interactions that take place between the ultrasound waves and the tissues of the breast, and highlights some of the instrumentation requirements.

HOW THE IMAGE IS FORMED

Sound Wave Interactions with Tissue

Formation of the ultrasound image begins with the transmission of a high frequency mechanical wave into and through the tissue. This energy wave is generated by a vibrating transducer, and is transmitted into the breast either directly through the skin (contact scanning) or by way of intervening water (water-path). As the wave propagates through the breast tissues, it may be reflected from flat surfaces, scattered from irregular surfaces, or absorbed by the friction of molecules colliding with one another as they transmit the ultrasound energy wave.

Recording Wave Interactions

The interactions of the ultrasound wave with the breast tissues eventuate in the return of a small amount of the original wave energy to the transducer. The vibration of the returning wave or echo induces a small voltage on the transducer surface, which is amplified in the unit's receiver. The strength of the wave and the time that elapses between the emission of the wave and the reception of the echo can be measured. Since the velocity of sound (1540m/sec) changes less than 8% when transmitted through tissue,[1] the elapsed time is used to compute the distance between the transducer and the reflecting tissue and, together with the strength of the wave, serves as the basis for the production of the breast image.

ULTRASOUND IMAGING COMPARED TO X-RAY IMAGING

It is possible to draw some comparisons between the physical principles that apply to x-ray mammography and those that apply to ultrasound mammography. Such comparison may be helpful to the physician who is experienced in x-ray mammography but not in ultrasound.

Focal Spot Versus Transducer

In some ways, the ultrasound transducer can be compared to the x-ray tube focal spot. Both are limited in their effects by trade-offs between resolution and tissue penetration. For example, just as a very small focal spot increases x-ray image resolution, a high frequency transducer increases ultrasound image resolution. However, the smaller the x-ray focal spot, the longer the exposure time that is required for adequate penetration of breast tissue; similarly, the higher the frequency of the sound wave, the more readily is it attenuated by breast tissue and the less its penetration of the breast.

Source-to-Skin Distance Versus Oil-Water Interface

A longer distance between the x-ray target and the breast has the beneficial effects of reducing scattered radiation and increasing the dimensions of the image. Similarly, ultrasound images are produced with a separation between the transducer and skin surface, thus decreasing reverberation artifacts (ring down) and increasing the field of view. Reverberation artifacts arise from mechanical waves generated in the transducer, which are reflected to and fro, appearing as dark bands that interfere with echoes from the adjacent skin and subcutaneous tissues. Other

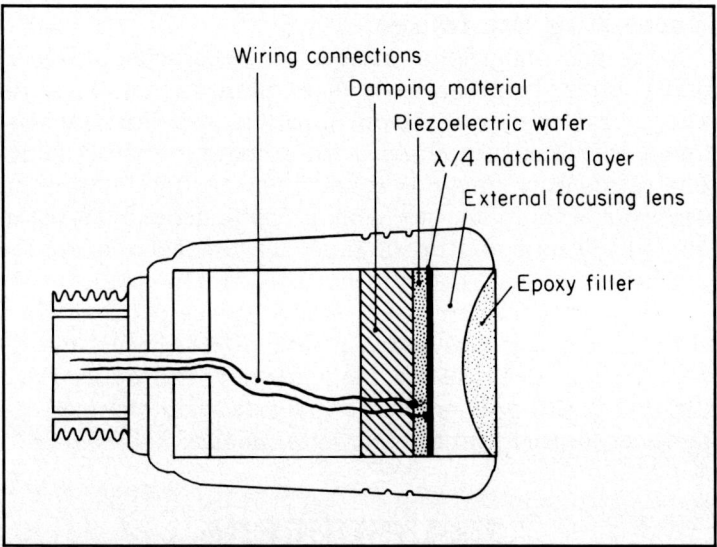

Figure 2-1. Transducer components.

artifacts result from the lack of a bell-shaped or Gaussian distribution of sound waves in the 1cm to 3cm field in front of the transducer, the so-called "near field." Because air does not transmit ultrasound adequately, the desired separation between the transducer and the breast surface must be achieved by the interposition of water, water-soluble acoustic gel, or oil.[2]

Amplifying the Image

The image detector in modern x-ray mammography is either a film-screen combination or an electronically charged xeromammographic selenium-coated aluminum plate. In film-screen mammography, the phosphor in the intensifying screen amplifies the x-ray photons by converting them to even more numerous light photons; in xeromammography, electrical field forces amplify the concentration of the powdered toner at the edges of a cancer and its calcifications. In ultrasound, the transducer, having recognized the reflected sound wave as mechanical energy, translates it into an electric voltage that is intensified by an electrical amplifier similar to that in a home stereophonic system.

Recording the Image

X-ray mammographic images are recorded on film or paper. Image contrast depends on many factors including x-ray target material, beam filtration, exposure factors, image receptor, and film or xeroradiographic processing. The ultrasound image is constructed in the digital scan converter, a computer-like memory component, and is based on calculations of the distance of the echo from the transducer and the amplitude of the signal. By "remembering" where the transducer was pointed when the echo was received, a plane of tissue echoes is constructed. Because the image memory is produced in a digital format, gray scale and magnification changes can be incorporated into the television image.

TRANSDUCERS

Basic Characteristics

The transducer is the key component of any ultrasound imaging system, since it is the most important determinant of image quality. Figure 2-1 diagrams a typical transducer. The transducer's piezoelectric wafer produces an ultrasonic wave when a voltage is applied to it and generates a voltage when vibrated by a mechanical wave. Ultrasound wafers are usually made from ceramic lead zirconate titanate (PZT), which is treated with heat and electricity to create piezoelectric properties. Recently, transducers constructed of layers of polyvinylidene fluoride (PVDF) have been used for high frequency wafers. Ultrasound waves can be produced at a variety of frequencies, depending on the thickness of the wafer. The thinner the wafer, the higher the center of frequency it will generate; for example, a 3.5MHz PZT wafer is 0.57mm thick, while a 7.5MHz wafer is 0.267mm thick (assuming that PZT4, a variation of PZT, is used for both wafers).[3]

The wafer is activated by a voltage pulse of 100-250V for 0.1μsec. The resultant mechanical pulse is transmitted into the patient, and is both reflected and scattered within the breast. The reflected waves return to the transducer where a voltage of between 0.1V and 100μV is generated by the wave striking the surface of the wafer.[4] Even if the wave traversed water instead of tissue, it would change along its passage because it is not generated by a vibrating point but by a vibrating surface about 1cm to 3cm in diameter. Indeed, each point on the surface of the wafer radiates a wavelet when the voltage activates it. These wavelets interact, re-enforcing and reducing the amplitude of the total wave as it travels from the wafer surface. At a distance from the wafer, called the focal zone, the individual waves begin to operate in unison. In the focal zone the re-enforced amplitude is at its maximum intensity and resolving power. The location of the focal zone depends on the frequency and diameter of the transducer wafer, as well as on the focusing method applied to the wafer. In the near zone, where the wavelets constructively and destructively interfere with each other, images show a heterogeneous texture that is dependent on the transducer and not the breast. After the wave passes beyond the focal zone and into the far field, its shape flattens and spreads so that a small lesion (0.6-1.2cm) may be imaged poorly or not at all (Figure 2-2).[5] With increasing diameter and frequency of the transducer, and for the same focal lens, the focal distance increases and the spreading of the beam in the far field becomes more gradual.

Focusing the Ultrasound Beam

Most breasts are 4cm to 12cm thick and can be compressed to a thickness of 2cm to 7cm. Therefore, the optimal focal zone of a hand-held transducer (such as a real-time unit with a 2cm water gap) is about 3cm to 6cm (Figure 2-3). Without a focusing lens, a 5MHz-2cm diameter transducer would have a focal point at 32.5cm. To obtain the desired focal zone an acoustic lens is placed on the transducer wafer. An acoustic lens of 4.9cm radius is needed to place the focal zone at a depth of 3cm to 6cm.[6] Unfortunately, the refocusing reduces the total area that is in sharp focus and results in rapid divergence of the beam, leading to elongation and loss of detail of the deeper breast structures (in the far field) (Figure 2-4).

An advantage of automated water path units is the long water offset built into the scanner, which allows for the

18 breast ultrasound

Figure 2-2. Effect of focal zone placement on shape of mass.

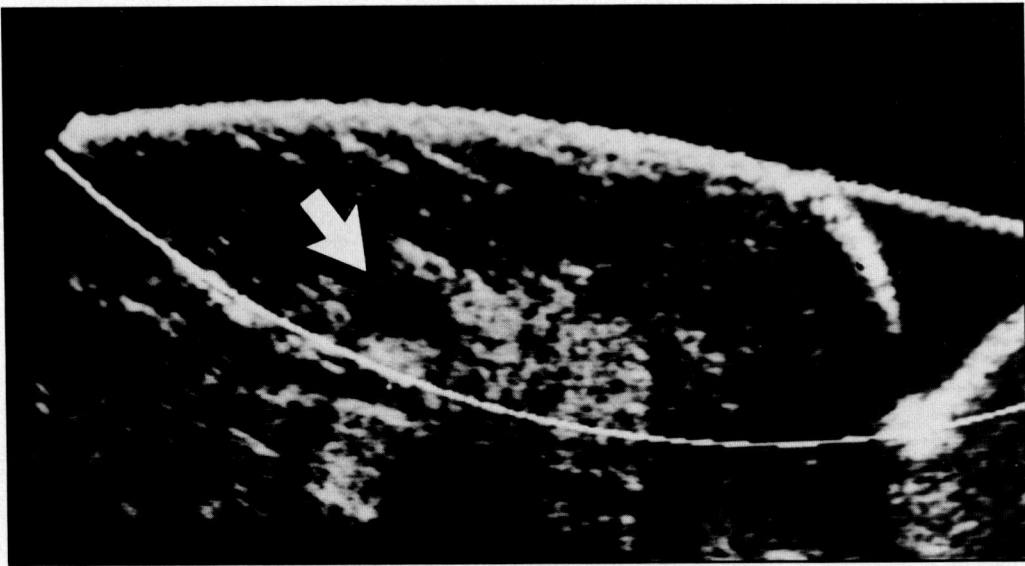

Figure 2-2A. Curved white line indicates focal zone. Round, smoothly marginated mass is indicated by arrow.

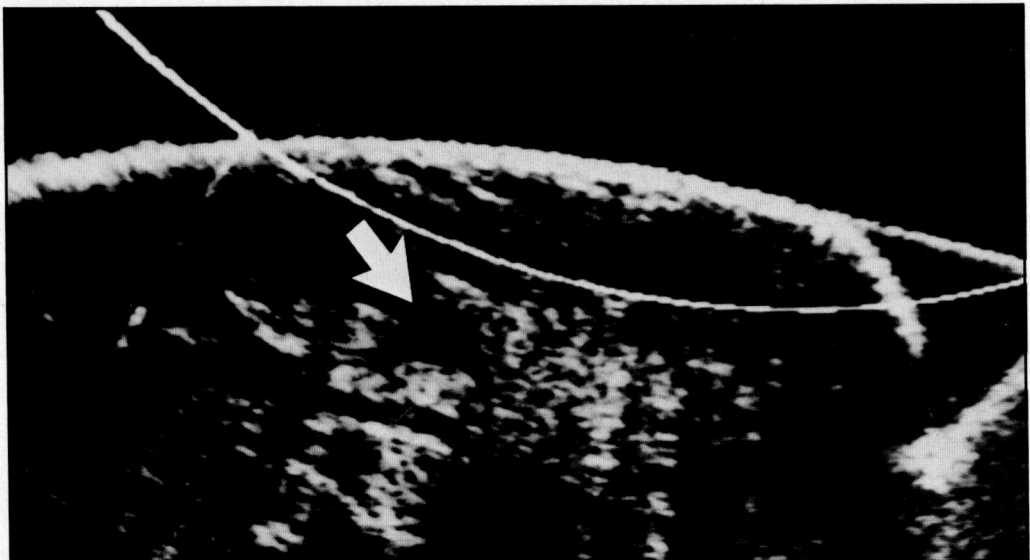

Figure 2-2B. When imaged in far field, mass appears irregular and slightly larger.

physics

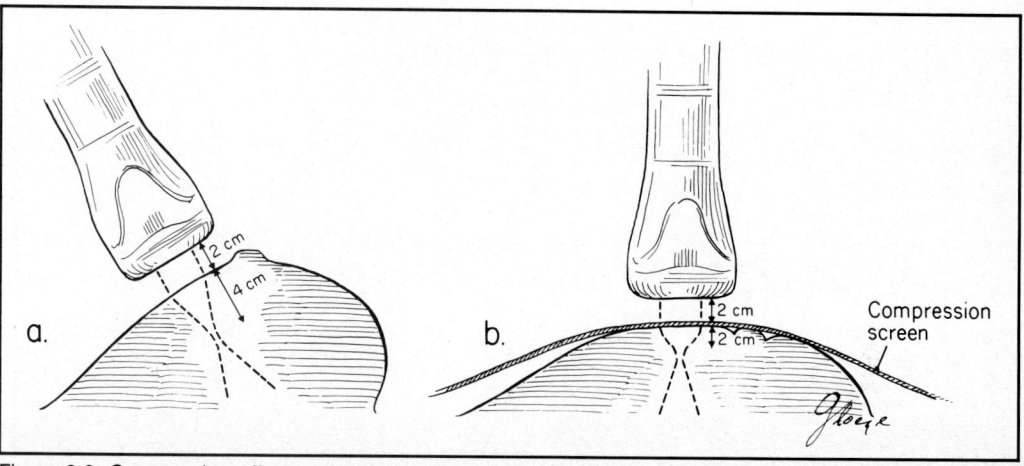

Figure 2-3. Compression affects selection of transducer. A. Noncompressed breast, 8cm thick. Optimal focal zone extends to depth of 4cm within breast. B. Compression, same breast, 4cm thick. Now optimal focal zone extends 2cm into breast.

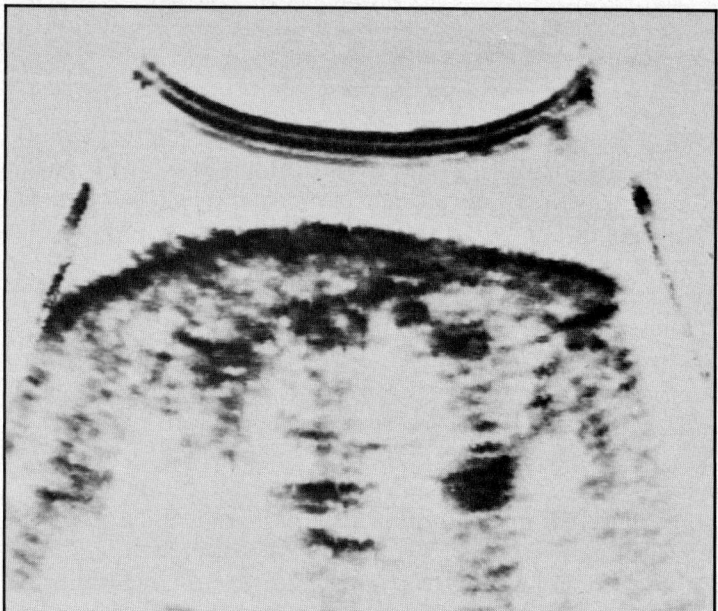

Figure 2-4. Effect of focal zone on image sharpness. Hand-held real-time examination with 7.5MHz transducer and 2cm water bag offset (in addition to 2cm offset within transducer). All structures are in the far zone, resulting in poor resolution from skin to chest wall. A 2cm mass in the center of the breast was not identified in the image.

20 *breast ultrasound*

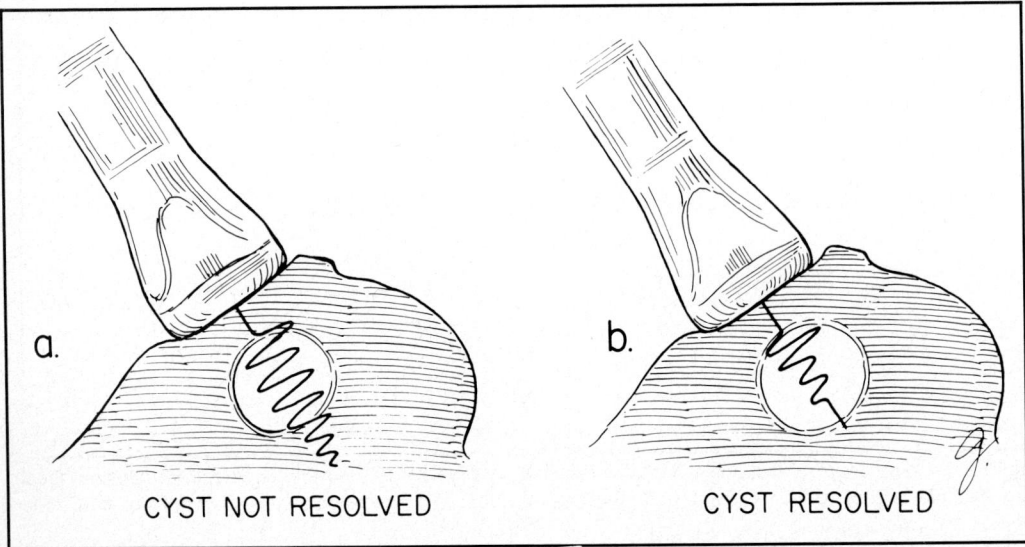

Figure 2-5. Axial resolution. A. The ultrasound pulse cycles are too numerous to resolve both the front and back wall of the mass. B. Shorter pulse (four cycles) resolves anterior and posterior walls.

use of a less-curved lens that produces less distortion of detail in the far field. Thus, a section of the whole breast and the adjacent chest wall structures can be clearly depicted in a single image.

Construction of the Transducer

The transducer must be constructed so that it does not continue to vibrate once the voltage pulse has been transmitted to the wafer. Continuation of the vibrations would interfere with the recognition of the reflected waves from breast structures (Figure 2-5). Therefore, the wafer is backed with a heavy material that dampens and absorbs outgoing waves that might otherwise be reflected from the back wall of the wafer. An acoustically matched layer of material attached to the front of the wafer prevents reverberations between the wafer and offset substance or focused transducer by computing the time it takes the wavelets to constructively interfere with each other if they were focused at a given distance.[7] This computation is based on an assumption that the velocity of sound in tissue is 1540m/sec. With this information, each small wafer in the array is fired with a delay so that its wavelet will arrive at the desired focal distance simultaneously with the others. The beam can also be directed to produce a patient. The matching layer also increases the intensity of the wave that is available for imaging, since more of the wave is transmitted into the breast. The material in the matching layer is designed specifically for a particular lens and for a particular offset substance; a water offset and an oil offset have different requirements. Because of these factors, the ultrasound pulse consists of three or four cycles as it enters the breast, and yields a resolution cell about 1mm in length, too long to permit the imaging of microcalcifications or objects less than 0.3cm in diameter.[2]

Motor Driven Transducers Versus Hand-Held Real-Time Transducers. The transducer can be moved manually across the breast (a form of hand-held real-time scanning called B-mode scanning); it may be moved back and forth by a motor, or a large series of tiny transducers may be electronically pulsed in sequence. The primary effort in the design of any motor driven transducer is to provide an even drive so that the scan lines are uniform and equally spaced. The heavier the transducer, the greater the tendency for uneven motion. Manufacturers may reduce the weight of a motor driven transducer by reducing the amount of damping material at its back. However, if the material in the layer in front of the transducer does not acoustically match the offset substance, axial resolution will be degraded. The problem of excessive transducer weight may also be avoided by leaving the transducer stationary and rocking an acoustic mirror in front of it, but images made by this method may lack adequate penetration and tend to contain artifactual echoes in anechoic regions. Another solution to uneven motion caused by a heavy transducer is to construct three transducers at 120° spacings about a motor and spin them continuously. With this method each transducer generates 1/3 of the sector image, and every third line in the sector is made by the same transducer. This requires precision matching and mounting of

22 breast ultrasound

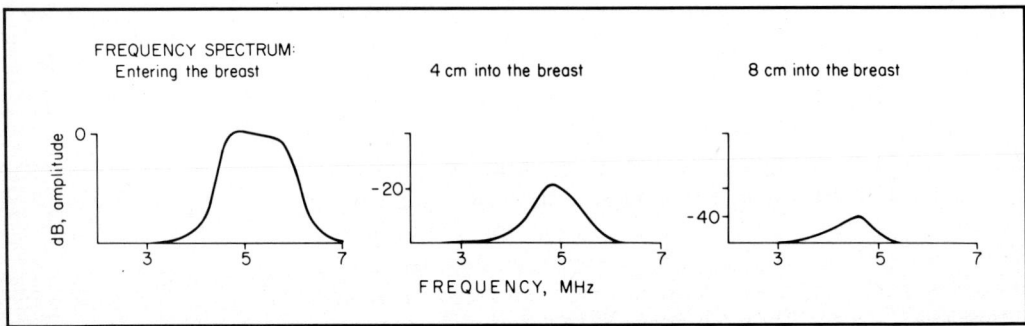

Figure 2-6. Attenuation of high frequency component of frequency spectrum. The entering wave contains a mixture of wave frequencies. More of the higher frequencies than the lower frequency waves are attenuated by tissue. After passing through 8cm of breast tissue (4cm into the breast and 4cm returning to the surface), the wave is diminished in amplitude and its peak frequency is lower than its initial peak frequency. This change continues at 8cm into breast tissue.

the transducers and doubles the cost of the transducer assembly.

Relatively inexpensive phased arrays of wafers recently have become available for breast imaging. These arrays simulate the wavelets emitted from a single large-diameter sectored image by similar delays in firing.[8] However, problems may occur because of the 8% variation in the velocity of sound in soft tissue and because the frequency emitted by the wafer is a mixture arranged around the center frequency, which is controlled by the wafer's thickness. For these reasons, the beam of some phased arrays may not be as precisely focused as that of motor driven transducers.

Frequency Band Width. A mixture of frequencies rather than a single frequency is generated by the piezoelectric wafer when it is activated by a short pulse of voltage. The wafer not only generates the outgoing wave, but dampens the returning wave to improve axial resolution. If the wave entering the breast has a center frequency of 5MHz, it could be expected to have 3.75MHz and 6.25MHz frequency wavelets. As the focal distance depends on the frequency of the transducer, the 3.75 and 6.25MHz frequencies will have different focusing components. Since high frequency waves are attenuated more rapidly than low frequency waves, the higher central frequencies in the spectrum of frequencies decrease as they travel through the breast (Figure 2-6). This causes the focal distance to shift progressively toward the transducer as the beam traverses an increasingly greater thickness of tissue.[9,10] For this reason, the larger the breast the deeper must the focal zone be placed.

ATTENUATION

Attenuation is the diminution in intensity of the ultrasound wave as it travels through the breast. Attenuation provides diagnostic information since various breast tissues have different attenuation values. Attenuation is due to two independent effects: absorption and scattering.

Absorption of Ultrasound in Tissue

While recent studies have indicated more complex interactions, the classical model of absorption is adequate for purposes of understanding the basic interactions that affect the ultrasound image. The classical explanation of ultrasound absorption is that it results from the heat generated by the friction between colliding molecules set in motion by the ultrasound wave. Thus, as the ultrasound frequency increases, the molecules move back and forth more rapidly, more collisions occur, more heat is generated, and absorption increases. The consistency or density of tissue affects absorption, since resistance to molecular movement will increase friction and so increase absorption. According to their progressively decreasing capacity for the absorption of ultrasound, the order of ranking for the tissues of the breast is: skin, glandular tissue or parenchyma, and fat.[11] In vitro studies of fresh mammalian tissue show that different tissues—including brain, heart, kidney, liver, tendon, and testis—have similar increases in attenuation and absorption as the ultrasound frequency increases[12]; therefore, the effects of relative attenuation remain whether a 3.5MHz transducer or a 7.5MHz transducer is used. Attenuation of ultrasound increases in all tissues with increasing frequency of the ultrasound wave. Breast cysts, benign tumors, and malignancies tend to have very different attenuation characteristics. A cyst absorbs less sound than the surrounding parenchymal tissue, so that enhancement of the echoes occurs behind the cyst. On the other hand, malignant tumors have been shown in vitro to absorb ultrasound two to three times greater than normal tissue or benign tumors.[13] This increased absorption of sound results in "shadowing" or an absence of echoes distal to the malignant lesion.

The Scattering of Ultrasound in Tissue

The scattering of ultrasound within tissue is largely determined by the size of the cells constituting the tissue and the spacing between them. Similarly, the characteristics of small echoes from within a lesion are determined by the consistency of the lesion. The quality of the information obtained regarding the scattering of sound waves, whether within tissue or a lesion, is highly dependent on the scanning equipment and the technique of scanning.

TIME GAIN COMPENSATION AND POWER

Time Gain Compensation

In the normal 6cm thick breast scanned at 5MHz, the returning ultrasound wave is attenuated to 0.001 of its original value. Imaging equipment compensates for this attenuation by amplifying the returning sound waves. The amount of amplification, or gain, must be greater for sound waves returning from the deepest portions of the breast since these will have undergone the greatest attenuation. The digital scan converter computes the depth of the tissue on the basis of the time it takes for the emitted signal to return to the transducer. The variable gain that is applied to the signal is therefore called time gain compensation (TGC). The TGC is usually adjusted by the technologist according to breast density and size, although one automatic breast scanner has a fixed TGC that cannot be adjusted. The TGC curve represents the increase in amplification with depth. Since the attenuation increases with increasing frequency, the slope of the TGC curve is steeper when higher frequency transducers are used.

A dense fibrocystic or dysplastic breast may require a steeper TGC curve than a breast that is only slightly glandular. However, if the TGC curve is too steep, the amplification capacity may be exhausted, causing the tissue posterior to the knee of the TGC curve (the break in the smooth line of the curve where the slope changes abruptly or is used up) to have inadequate amplification. This may prohibit the recording of such valuable diagnostic information as shadowing or enhancement of echoes behind masses.

Power

Called variously "sonic intensity," "output power," "percent power," or even "dB" on the consoles of some units, power refers to the amount of voltage applied to the transducer to produce the mechanical wave that enters the patient. Like the watts emitted by a radio broadcasting station, the power affects the distance that the wave travels in the breast before it is completely attenuated. However, if the power is too great the echoes returning from the near field will saturate the amplifier, producing an excessively bright image without texture or gray level variation. Furthermore, all the dampened cycles in the short pulse of ultrasound emitted by the transducer will be amplified, so that axial resolution will be degraded. For these reasons technologists are usually advised to keep the power as low as possible consistent with adequate penetration of the breast to the chest wall. If the image shows returning echoes but anatomic details cannot be seen in the far field, the power is probably too high and the image deep in the breast is more than likely to represent mere noise.

Artifacts Due to Inappropriate TGC and Power

If the TGC is set correctly, simple cysts will manifest an absence of interior echoes, fat will show a few low level echoes, and a fibroadenoma will show numerous

26 breast ultrasound

Figure 2-7. Cyst.

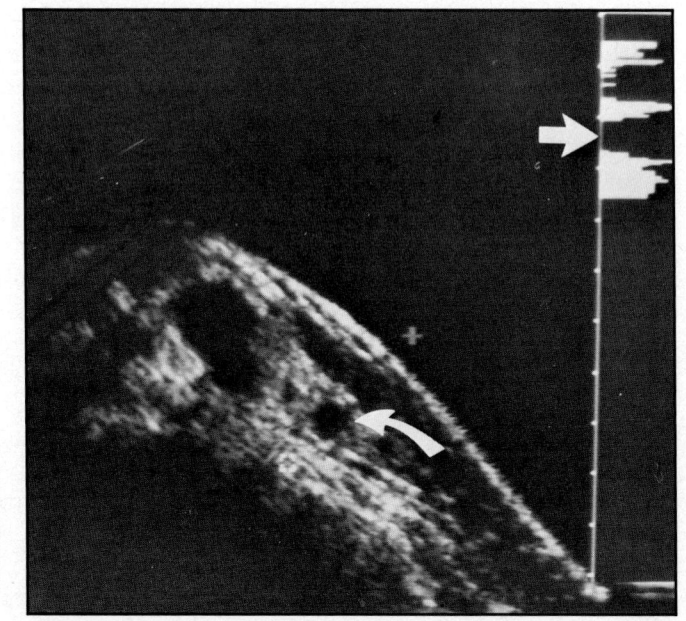

Figure 2-7A. Ultrasound breast image shows a small cyst adjacent to chest wall (curved arrow). Note the homogeneous echoes in the A-line at the level of the subcutaneous fat, and the absence of echoes in the cyst (arrow).

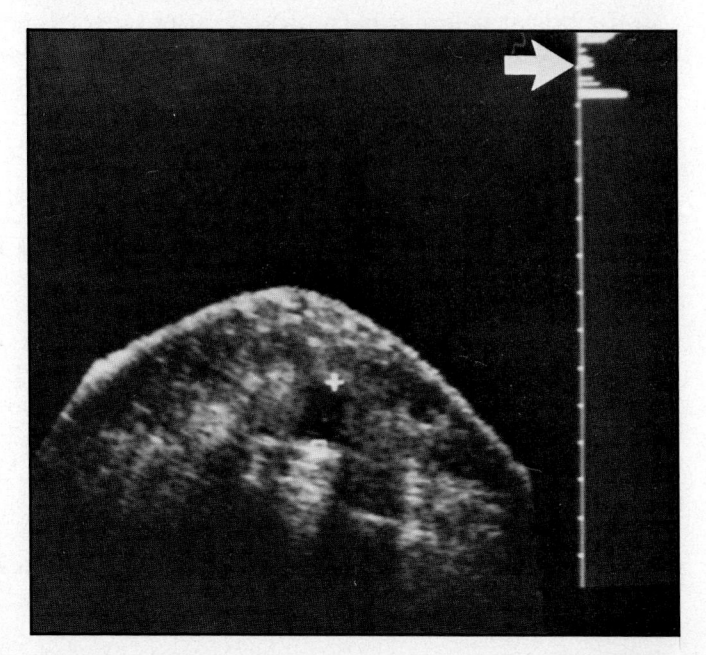

Figure 2-7B. Solid mass. Heterogeneous interior echoes in a solid tumor with posterior enhancement. The A-line confirms the low amplitude echoes within the mass (arrow).

homogeneous internal echoes of moderate amplitude (Figure 2-7). An inappropriate TGC can result in artifactual echoes and shadows (Figure 2-8). A very steep TGC curve will lead to a depletion of amplification capabilities within the first few centimeters of tissue and an absence of echoes in the deeper tissue. Too much power can result in apparent echoes within a cyst, while too little power may cause a solid mass to appear anechoic simulating a cyst (Figure 2-9).

REFLECTION AND REFRACTION

The principles of energy reflection and refraction that apply to ultrasound imaging may have important effects on the appearance of masses. Reflection is the return of sound waves from a surface. Refraction is the deflection of a sound wave from its straight path as it passes obliquely from one medium into another when the velocities of the mediums differ.

Ultrasonic Impedance

Ultrasound impedance is the property of tissue that controls the amount of reflection of the ultrasound wave. Because masses and tissue interfaces within the breast reflect less than 10% of the ultrasound wave, reflection does not contribute to as great a loss of ultrasound energy as attenuation. Strong reflections of sound may occur at a hard surface, such as the capsule or boundary of a mass, or at the interface between two tissues of differing acoustic impedance such as the junction between subcutaneous fat and parenchyma. The interface between tissues can be appreciated only when they have a different impedance. Ultrasonic impedance depends on tissue density and elasticity (or velocity). The breast usually has many reflecting surfaces since fat (impedance of 1.41 Rayls) separates layers of glandular tissue (impedance of 1.63 Rayls) throughout its extent. Although the capsule of a cyst is too thin to resolve with most ultrasound instruments, the interface between the surrounding tissue and the cyst capsule/fluid shows up clearly. Since a solid tumor is usually denser

28 breast ultrasound

Figure 2-8. Time gain compensation curves.

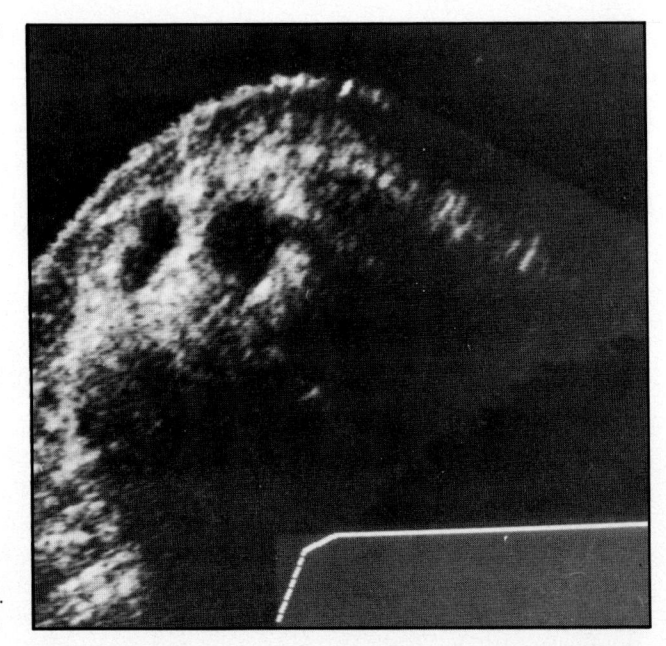

Figure 2-8A. TGC curve too steep. Artifactual echoes within cysts (arrows).

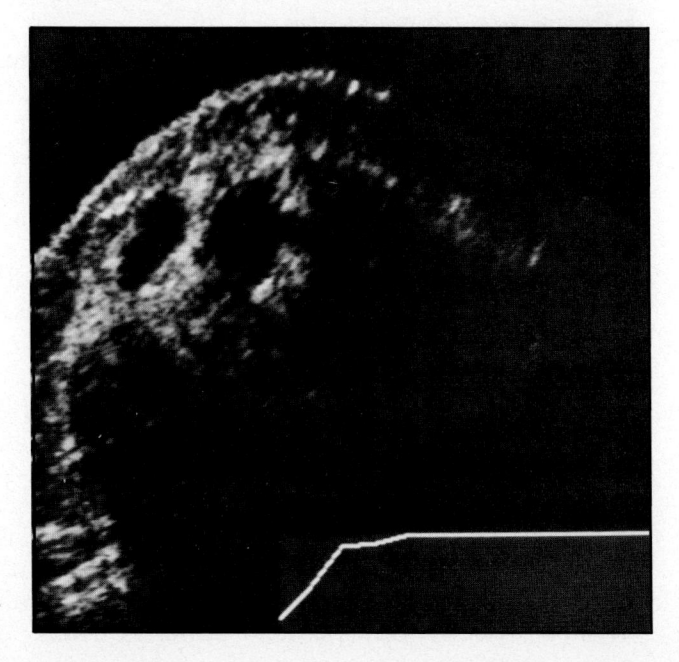

Figure 2-8B. TGC curve less steep. Absence of artifactual internal echoes.

physics   29

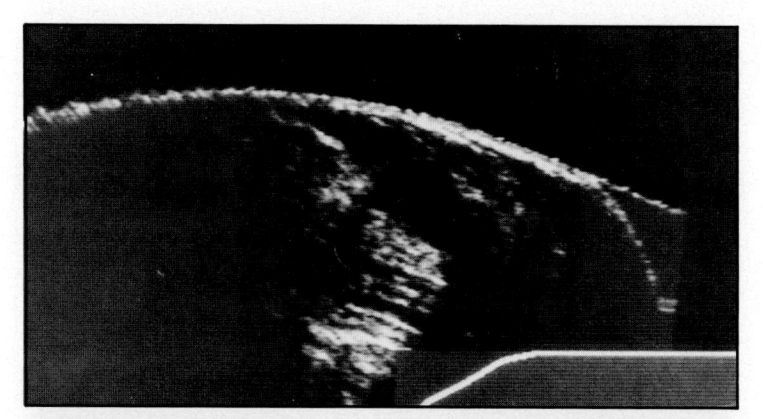

Figure 2-9. Power.

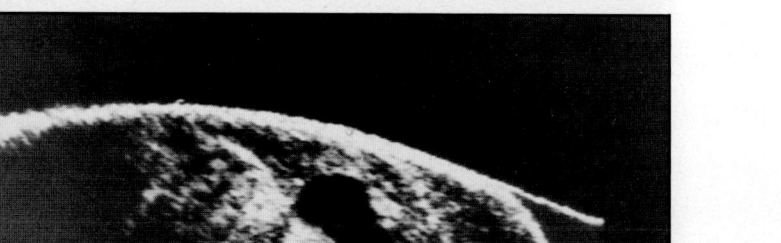

Figure 2-9A. Insufficient power to depict cyst.

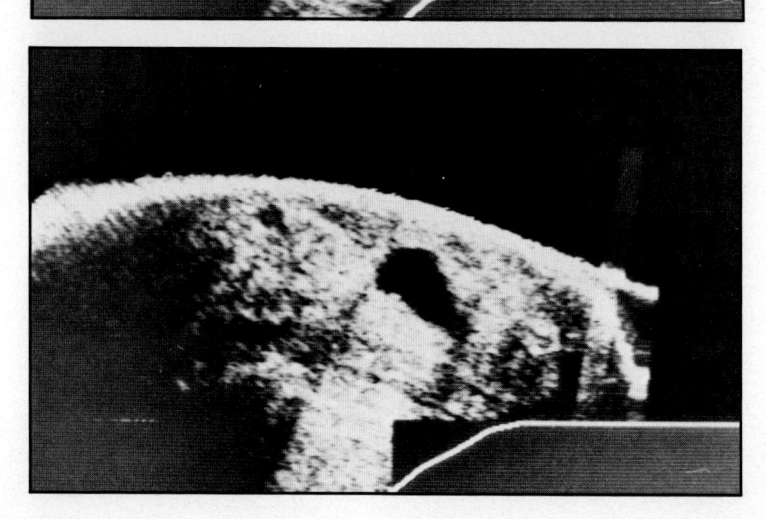

Figure 2-9B. Greater power setting confirms absence of internal echoes and enhancement of distal echoes.

Figure 2-9C. Too much power results in an excessively bright image with inadequate grey level texture.

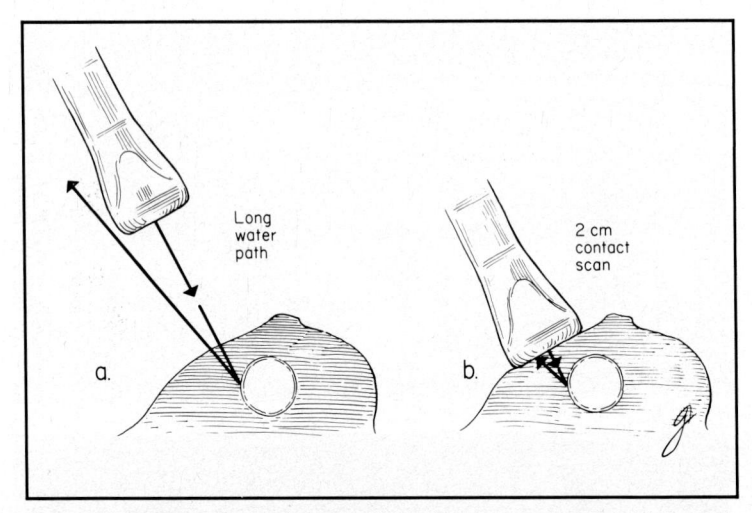

Figure 2-10. Effect of transducer to object distance on depiction of mass. A. Water path scan. Transducer misses returning wave. B. Hand-held real-time unit. Short distance results in return of more reflected waves from curved boundary of object.

and less elastic than the surrounding tissue, the boundaries between the two reflect the ultrasound wave, making the tumor visible in the image.

Reflection from Curved Edges

Since an interface can be visualized only if the reflected waves reach the transducer, interfaces that are not parallel to the transducer face will be poorly imaged. The fall in intensity will be directly proportional to the diameter of the transducer, the degree of interface curvature, and the distance from the transducer (Figure 2-10). Hand-held instruments with a short distance between the breast and the transducer will image the boundaries of curved lesions more completely than automated units with a large water offset between the transducer and the breast.

Refraction and Critical Angle

Refraction occurs where there is a change in velocity of sound transmission between two adjacent tissues, and the boundary between the tissues is slanted with respect to

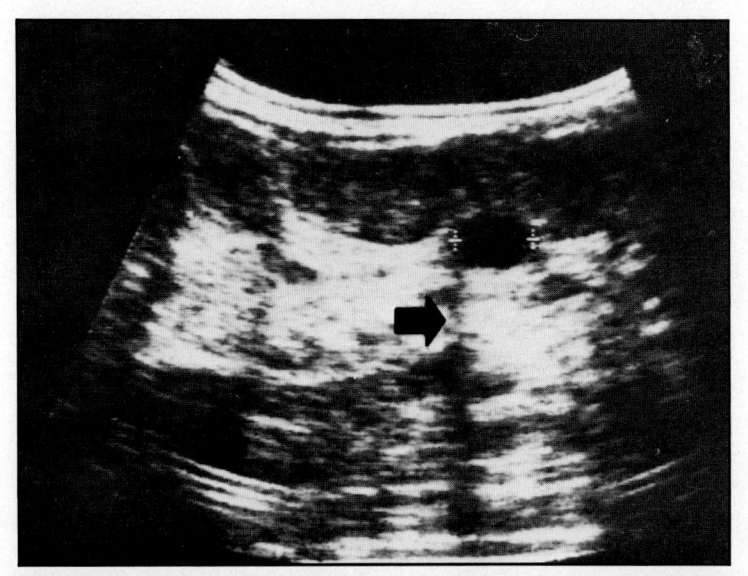

Figure 2-11. The shadows (arrow) distal to the sides of the cyst are due to critical angle refraction, and not gradually weakening reflection.

the transducer face. When two tissues have the same impedance but different velocities, the beam may be refracted but not reflected. In ultrasound, unlike optics, the gradual fading of the reflected wave from boundaries at the edges of a round lesion differs from the abrupt loss of lateral boundaries due to critical angle refraction. Refraction is used when focusing the ultrasound beam, since the lens attached to the piezoelectric wafer in the transducer bends the beam toward the desired focal distance in soft tissue. However, the beam refracts away from the center of a cyst when it strikes the curved edge of the cyst capsule. As the curve increases, the refraction eventually becomes so acute that no ultrasound waves can enter the cyst, and acoustic shadowing occurs distal to the lateral walls of the cyst (Figure 2-11). Automated scanners with a water offset produce acoustic shadows at the round medial and lateral surfaces of the breast when the breast curvature is greater than 50° relative to the incident ultrasound beam.[14] This is the critical angle at which all of the sound is refracted.

References

1. McDicken WN: Diagnostic Ultrasonics: Principles and Use of Instruments. New York: John Wiley and Sons, 1981, pp 56, 68.

2. Fornage BD, Touche DH, Rifkin MD: Small-parts real time sonography: A new "water path." J Ultrasound Med 3:355-358, 1984.

3. Wells PNT: Biomedical Ultrasonics. San Francisco: Academic Press, 1977, p 52.

4. Erickson KR, Fry FJ, Jones JP: Ultrasound in medicine. A review. IEEE Trans Sonics and Ultras SU-21:144-170, 1974.

5. Jaffe CC, Taylor JW: The clinical impact of ultrasonic beam focussing patterns. Radiology 131:469-472, 1979.

6. Kossoff G: Analysis of focusing action of spherically curved transducers. Ultrasound in Med and Biol 5:359-365, 1979.

7. Iinuma K, Kidokorot, Ogura I, et al: High resolution electronic-linear scanning ultrasonic diagnostic equipment. Ultrasound in Med and Biol 5:51-59, 1979.

8. Gatzke RD, Fearnside JT, Karp SM: Electronic scanner for a phased-array ultrasound transducer. Hewlett-Packard Journal 34.12:13-20, 1983.

9. Banjavic RA: Ultrasonic pulse-echo beam width and axial response approximations for clinical broadband focused transducers. Ultrasound in Med and Biol 7:63-71, 1981.

10. Zagzebski JA, Banjavic RA, Madsen EL, et al: Focused transducer beams in tissue-mimicking material. JCU 10:159-166, 1982.

11. O'Brien WD: The role of collagen in determining ultrasonic propagation properties in tissue, *In* Kessler LW (ed): Acoustic Holography, vol 7. New York: Plenum Press, 1977, p 37.

12. Goss SA, Fizzel LA, Dunn F: Ultrasonic absorption and attenuation in mammalian tissues. Ultrasound in Med and Biol 5:181-186, 1979.

13. Calderon C, Vilkomerson D, Mezrich R, et al: Differences in the attenuation of ultrasound by normal, benign and malignant breast tissue. JCU 4:249-254, 1976.

14. Kossoff G, Jellins J: The physics of breast echography. Seminars in Ultrasound 3:5-12, 1982.

CHAPTER 3

Instrumentation and Technique

INTRODUCTION

The interpretation of ultrasound examinations requires a knowledge of the basic mechanisms involved in making the image. Unlike x-ray mammography, in which the x-ray technologist actually performs the examination, if a real-time ultrasound unit with a hand-held transducer is used it is the physician who most often performs the examination. If the sonogram is an automated one of the whole breast, it is usually performed by the technologist; the physician subsequently reviews 15 to 30 polaroid or multiformatted films or hundreds of frames on videotape in order to visualize the dynamics involved in the formation of the image, an appreciation of which will enhance his or her diagnostic acumen.

This chapter describes how the ultrasound image is generated and compares features of general units and dedicated breast units. Practical aspects of performing the examination, such as positioning and compression, are also discussed.

SIGNAL PROCESSING

Creating an ultrasound breast image involves several steps that begin after the returning sound wave is detected by the transducer. Time gain compensation (TGC) takes into account the attenuation of the wave by the breast tissues. The receiver amplifies and filters the returning signal. The signal must then be put into digital form so that it can be stored in the computer memory.

TGC Regulation

Time gain compensation for attenuation of the sound wave through the breast depends primarily on the TGC beginning depth, the initial compensation for skin, the slope (higher frequencies require a steeper slope), and the total depth.

Some ultrasound units control these parameters with dials labeled "slope start," "near gain," "slope," and "far gain," and display the TGC curve on the TV monitor to inform the technologist of the effect of these settings on the breast image. Other machines use sliders that control the TGC at various depths along the path of the ultrasound wave; for example, sliders 2 and 3 may control the TGC at depths of 4cm and 6cm respectively. If the sliders that control the TGC are at uneven divisions of breast tissue depth, the TGC curve should be displayed on the TV monitor.

Receivers

The reflected signal is relatively weak, with a large number of frequencies admixed with the center frequency. Some ultrasound units amplify the returning signal before the TGC is applied, while others consider this initial amplification to be the first stage of the TGC. The mixture of frequencies must be preserved after amplification, since it allows the identification of short voltage pulses representing the edges of ducts and small lesions. Because a wide bandwidth limits the amount of amplification that can be applied by a single amplifier, a cascade of amplifiers is used, which increases not only the diagnostic information but also the noise. Since filtration of this noise may also remove the high frequency signals needed for good resolution, some manufacturers logarithmically amplify (log-amp) the signals when they are first received. The log-amp technique selectively amplifies low amplitude signals (and noise) more than medium and high amplitude signals. This preliminary logarithmic amplification may create echoes in anechoic structures such as cysts, may cause shadows behind tumors, and may reduce the echo enhancement distal to cysts. Flaws in the design of transducers and receivers account for more than 70% of the untoward variations in image quality.

Filtration

Some units filter out those returning signal frequencies that are either too high or too low to be within the available bandwidth of the transducer. This is exemplified in a dial on Philips units that acts to filter out specific bandwidths of frequencies.

Digitization

After amplification and filtration, the signal is digitized for storage in the computer memory, termed the digital scan converter (DSC). The memory size, modulation method, magnification factor, and highest received frequency determine the sampling rate of the digitizer. Recent electronic innovations have made practical the high sampling rate required by a high frequency 7.5MHz transducer. Numerous methods are available to process the signal and each of these alters the resulting image.[1] Most methods for digitization use only the signal amplitude[2] and do not consider the phase changes in the reflected sound wave. A unit that produces an image based on both amplitude and phase changes of the returning wave is currently being evaluated at several institutions.

Gray Level, Dynamic Range, Contrast. The gray level values or steps assigned during digitization may affect the low level signals from hypoechoic tissue such as fat. If 15 gray levels are available for the final image (four bits would give 16 gray levels, but one bit is usually reserved for labeling) and the voltage range of the amplified signal is 0.01V to 5V, a voltage could be assigned ranging from 0.01V to 0.34V to the first gray level, 0.341V to 0.674V to the second gray level, etc. Each 0.333V increase would be assigned to the next consecutive gray level. This linear mapping produces an acceptable ultrasound image if the receiver log-amplifies the initial signal. If a linear amplifier is used, the image shows only anatomical boundaries; texture is entirely absent. Some units log-amplify the initial signal and assign a logarithmic gray level map as the signal is digitized. The curve of the gray level map influences contrast and lesion detectability (Figure 3-1). Similarly, a change in the voltage range that is assigned to the various gray levels will alter the gray scale in the image. A gray scale map in the 0.01V to 5V range will not include very fine echoes. If the range is limited to 0.01V to 2V, thus deleting the echoes between 2V and 5V, each gray level step represents 0.142V and more textures are displayed. This remapping limits the dynamic range but increases the contrast.

38 breast ultrasound

Figure 3-1. Effect of gray level map. Different postprocessing gray level maps account for differences in depiction of same solid mass (arrow) in 3-1A and B. Pathologic diagnosis: fibroadenoma.

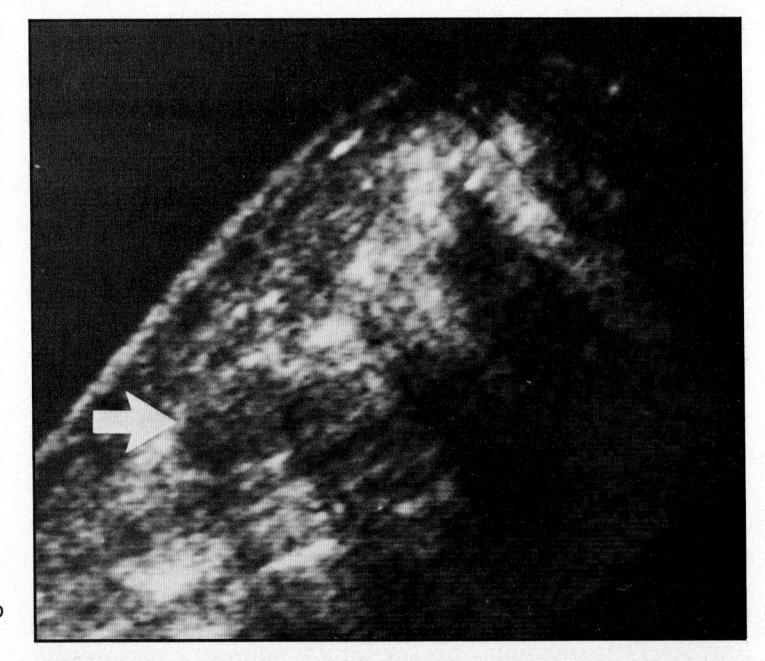

Figure 3-1A. Mass is difficult to perceive.

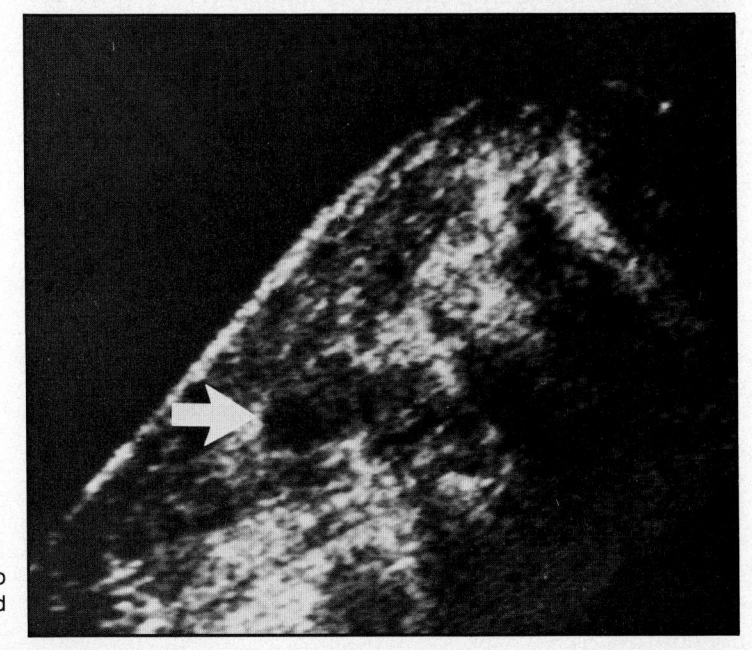

Figure 3-1B. Mass appears to have more distinct margin and fewer internal echoes.

Increasing the number of gray levels does not improve contrast, but may make low level echoes representing texture more subtle and pleasing. Some units offer the option of changing the gray level assignments after scanning ("postprocessing"). After the signal has been digitized according to some sort of "preprocessing" scheme, the memory cells' gray level steps can be changed again when the image is displayed on the TV monitor. Postprocessing allows windowing and other gray level manipulations, but it is only helpful if more than 16 gray levels have been assigned at digitization.

The Display Mode. Whether one favors black echoes on a white background or white echoes on a black background is a matter of personal preference. White on black seems to enhance the detection of lesions and the visualization of echoes within masses, and is preferred by most ultrasonographers.[3] Images using either mode are presented throughout this book.

Storage Assignment. Each line of ultrasound emitted from the transducer is assumed to be straight. Even if refraction occurs, the reflected signal is refracted back to its original path. The instrumentation "knows" the direction of the path of ultrasound because the motor drive (or phasing in an electrically driven array) is calibrated with a DSC memory storage table that allows the digitized signals from the returning ultrasound wave to be placed in their proper locations. All hand-held real-time units and all but one automated unit erase the computer memory before filling it with new information. The Ausonics automated unit gray level assignment is dependent on the previous gray level assignment in computer memory when two or more transducers simultaneously scan the same tissue (compound scanning).

If the lines emitted from the transducer are not close enough and the memory cells are not all filled, moire wave patterns may distort the image. For this reason, the empty memory cells are usually filled with data interpolated from adjacent digitized ultrasound signals.[4]

HAND-HELD REAL-TIME INSTRUMENTATION

Real-time units, whether mechanical or electrical, send a series of ultrasound pulses into the breast in a predictable manner so that the returning echoes can be mapped into an image. A "frame" is the series of pulses that make one image, and the "frame rate" is the speed at which the individual images are formed. A trade-off occurs between tissue depth, frame rate, and the number of pulses for each image. Since the required frame rate and depth are relatively modest for breast imaging, the number of pulses (or lines) per image can be maximized.

For hand-held instruments, the operator electronically labels the image according to the breast quadrant being scanned; whole-breast automated units perform this function automatically. Real-time, rather than B-mode static scanning, is preferred for breast imaging because the rapid display of adjacent slices provides the operator with a three-dimensional appreciation of the anatomy, even at 15 frames/sec.

Mechanical Units

General purpose real-time units with mechanically moving transducers are currently priced between $22,000 and $60,000. For breast imaging, 5 to 7.5MHz transducers with a 1cm to 3cm focal zone should be used. A 1cm to 3cm fluid offset may be offered for breast imaging with high frequency transducers, but a thicker offset is more satisfactory since the water-skin interface is likely to cause reverberation artifacts at less than 3cm depth. The following test can be used to compare the imaging characteristics of different units for low level signals.

Practical Test for Breast Imaging

Cut a natural (not synthetic) sponge in half so that each half is no more than 1cm thick. Submerge both slices in a tank of hot water, squeezing them to remove all air bubbles. Allow the water and sponge to spontaneously degas for at least an hour. Then fill a small balloon or condom with water and, after allowing a small amount of air to be entrapped, tie off the orifice. Insert the balloon between the two sponges in the water tank, and compress the sponges so that the whole sandwich is less than 5cm thick. (For stability, it may help to squeeze the sandwich into a hot water-filled half-gallon milk carton from which the top has been removed; the bottom sponge should be adjacent to the floor of the carton; then place this entire assemblage into the water tank). Scan across the top sponge and observe the enhancement behind the water-filled balloon, the shadow of the air bubble (if the scan includes that region), and the acoustic fill-in of the image of the water-filled portion of the balloon when power or TGC is increased. It should be possible to completely image the sponge above and the one below the balloon without increasing power or TGC to the extent that filling-in occurs in the image of the bladder. Observe any reverberation effects from the fluid offset, and change them by increasing the amount of water in the container above the top sponge. The distance between the transducer and offset membrane image will equal the distance between the offset membrane and the first reverberation.

Focal Zone Adjustment. When scanning a breast that contains a superficial mass, it may be necessary to increase the offset with a water bag to bring the focal zone closer to the lesion. Black lines in the image may represent air trapped in the water bag or too little gel between the offset and breast. Without a water offset, beam patterns in the near field, which vary greatly in intensity about the beam axis, will create artifacts and, more importantly, echoes in anechoic lesions.

Correct adjustment of the focal zone is critical when evaluating a small lesion. If too much of a water offset is used, the lesion will be imaged by the far field of the transducer, and distal enhancement or shadowing may be missing.[5]

Mechanical Real-Time Artifacts

Besides reverberations from the fluid offset, mechanical

units can, depending on their construction, produce several other artifacts:

Frame Jump. This artifact can occur in two ways: if the frame is not reformed at each sweep of the transducer but only every other line of the frame is changed, the image may contain information from the previous position of the transducer, or if the motor is not synchronized with the DSC memory storage table, the sweep from right to left may not be the same as the sweep from left to right. This causes a blurring in the interlaced frame, or a jumping between frames when each frame is refreshed at each sweep of the transducer.

Range Ambiguity. When a high frame is used to image a large breast containing large cysts, a shimmer in the anechoic lesions is produced. This artifact, which is not usually encountered in breast imaging, can be removed by reducing the frame rate. The shimmer is the result of ultrasound echoes returning from a previous scan line during the "listening" period of the present scan line.

Side Lobes. All transducers have low beam amplitude patterns that angle out to the side of the on-axis beam. The reflections from these skewed beams take longer to return to the transducer because they travel in a diagonal rather than a direct path. Therefore, their reflectors in the breast appear deeper than their actual location. When this occurs in the center of a cyst, it may cause the cyst to be interpreted as a solid lesion. A test using the sandwich of sponges and water-filled balloon should identify a unit whose log amplifier causes these side lobes to be imaged.

Lateral Measurement. Some mechanical sectors may slow down at the end of the sector, when they are preparing to reverse direction. If this speed change is not incorporated into the DSC memory storage table, a lateral measurement made at the edge of the sector (of large superficial lesions, for instance) will be inaccurate.[6] This artifact is machine-dependent and can be identified by imaging a thread test object placed across the sector (Figure 3-2A). If the thread

instrumentation and technique **43**

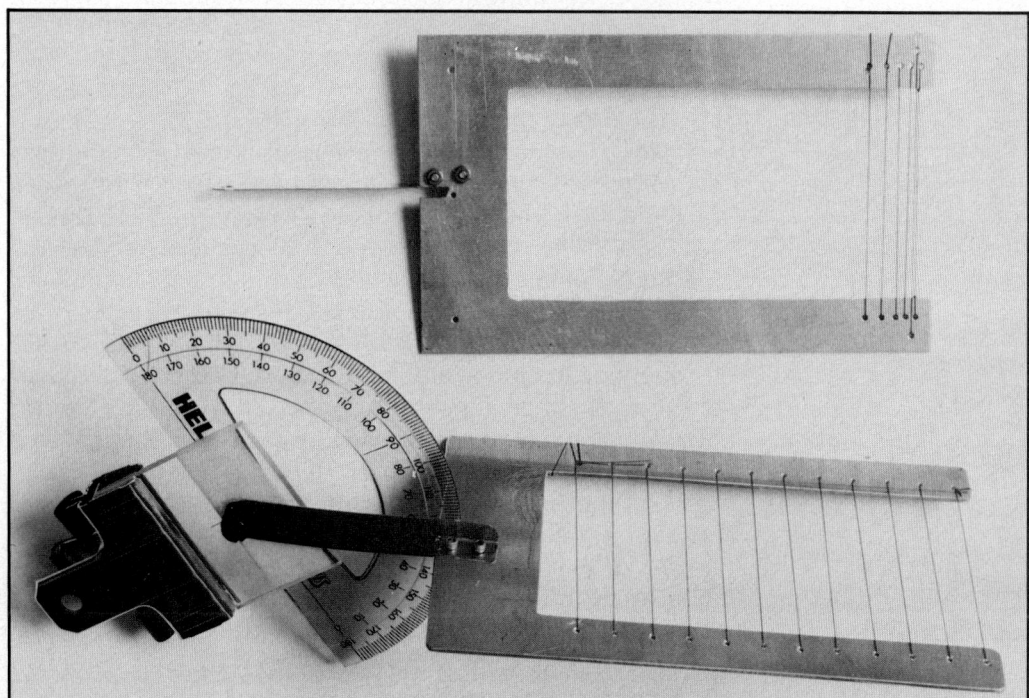

Figure 3-2. Quality control: Calibration of sector storage in real-time units.

Figure 3-2A. Thread test objects shown here are homemade from drafting materials and fishing filament.

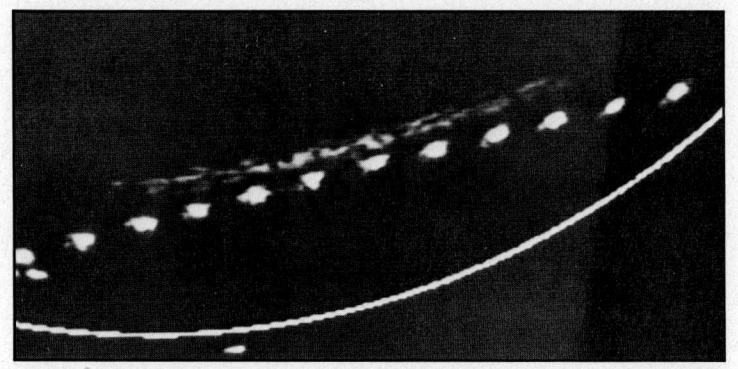

Figure 3-2B. Threads scanned across sector to test for mechanical storage errors at edges. Each white flash represents one thread. Scan shows good memory allocation at edges of sector.

images bend down at the sides of the sector, the decrease in motor speed has not been incorporated into the DSC storage algorithm (Figure 3-2B).

Phased Array Units

These units are relatively new and can range from those dedicated to breast imaging to multi-purpose units with variable focal zones. Their costs range from $16,000 to $120,000. When the focal zone can be modified by changing the delays of the signals, water offsets to adjust the focal zone are not needed. For breast imaging, where only a limited focal zone is useful, units that are "in focus" throughout the range of imaging are not required. Because of the wide range of tissues intermixed within the breast, phased arrays may not provide as focused an image as a mechanical unit for a large heterogeneous breast. A comparison between two array units, a mechanical unit and an automated whole breast unit, which all image the breast of a young woman with a large solid tumor, is illustrated in Figure 3-3.

Slice Thickness. Because the phased array elements are rectangular rather than circular, the lateral resolution will be different in the slice thickness direction.[7] Furthermore, the slice thickness direction cannot be focused by phasing, and so relies on an external focusing lens with a fixed focus. Since a general purpose unit may have the slice thickness focus deeper than required for breast imaging, it is important to learn from the manufacturer where this focus occurs and how deep the slice is "in focus." Small cysts imaged outside of the slice thickness focal range, even when they are in the phased array lateral focal range, may be filled in by the partial volume effect.

Phased Array Artifacts. Besides slice thickness effects, two other artifacts are unique to phased arrays and will affect the diagnostic quality of the breast images:

Grating Lobes. These produce diagonal filaments off the edges of anechoic lesions and may masquerade as a septum.

Figure 3-3. Four images of breast of 28-year-old woman. Large solid mass is present (arrows).

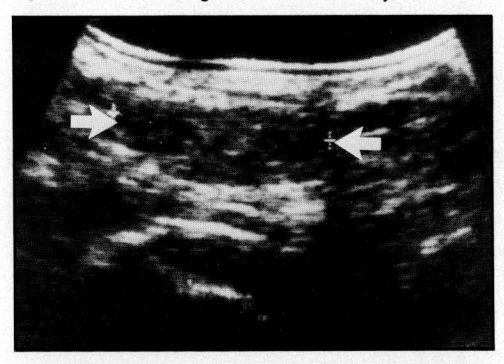

Figure 3-3A. Philips 3000 mechanical sector, 7.5MHz.

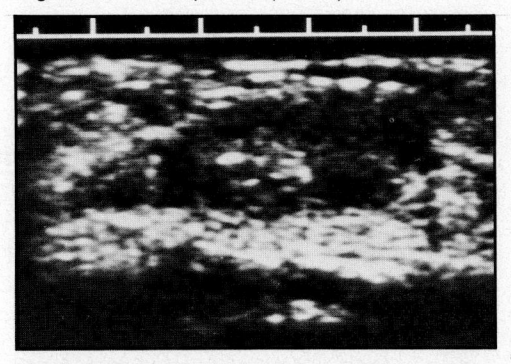

Figure 3-3B. Acuson phased array, 5MHz.

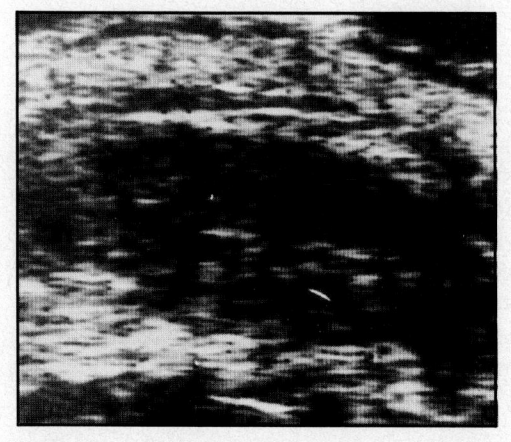

Figure 3-3C. Picker microview, 10MHz linear array with a water offset.

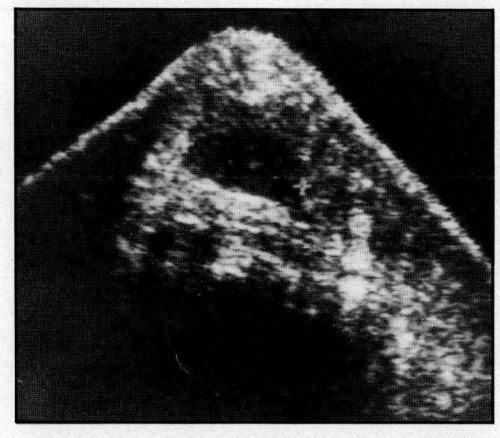

Figure 3-3D. Ausonics dedicated breast scanner, 4.5MHz. The pathologic diagnosis was fibroadenoma.

Grating lobes result from poorly designed arrays. If the separation between transducer element centers is kept to less than a wavelength, grating lobes will not affect the image.

Failed elements. Dark streaks that do not disappear when more acoustic gel is placed between the breast and transducer are probably caused by broken or missing array elements. These are particularly noticeable in a linear array but can also be seen in a phased array, where the failed element contributes to poor focusing.

Real-Time Scanning Techniques

Patient Positioning. The patient is placed supine and then slightly rotated by means of a towel behind her back on the side of the breast being scanned. The nipple should be centered, the back arched, and the ipsilateral arm comfortably abducted to help spread out the breast and allow greater access to the axillary tail.

Palpable Lumps, or Area Scans. For a palpable lump, the sonographer also obtains several images of the identical region of the contralateral normal breast. Once optimal instrument parameters have been established for the normal breast, the breast containing the palpable lump is scanned with the same parameters, in several planes, with some planes perpendicular to each other. The diameter of the mass is measured at its maximum in two perpendicular planes. While area scans can often differentiate between a solid and cystic lesion, it is usually better to survey both breasts carefully and methodically to avoid missing a nonpalpable lesion and to establish an ultrasonic baseline for future examinations. If the breast is predominantly fatty, then the survey can be omitted, since it will usually be nondiagnostic.

Breast Survey Techniques. Because most breasts are soft, pressure from the transducer will deform them, making the anatomical position difficult to record. For this reason, an abundance of acoustic gel (rather than oil, which tends to run off) and a light touch by the sonographer are needed. However, large breasts sometimes require more compression with the transducer in order to penetrate to the chest wall. A small breast can be imaged in eight slices; the first four are taken with the transducer placed at 12:00, 3:00, 6:00 and 9:00. The remaining four slices are made with the transducer placed halfway between the nipple and the edge of the breast, so that the four quadrants are

instrumentation and technique 47

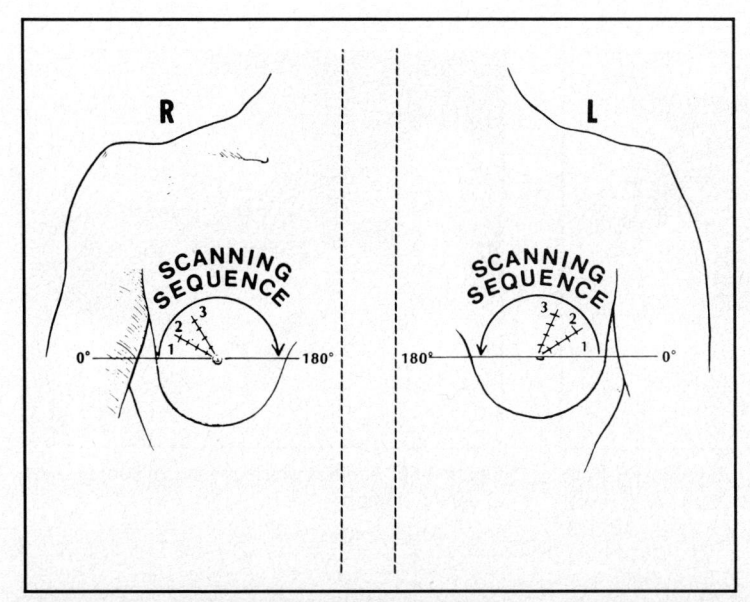

Figure 3-4. Breast examination with a hand-held transducer requires methodical scanning pattern. Although not illustrated here, ipsilateral arm should ideally be abducted to help spread out breast and allow greater access to axillary tail. From Baum: JUM 2:363, 1983.

imaged in planes perpendicular to the first four planes. The transducer can be rocked to cover the breast volume between the labelled planes. When scanning larger breasts, follow this general plan, but increase the first four slices to six (at 12:00, 2:00, 4:00, 6:00, 8:00 and 10:00) and make several slices between each pie shaped wedge (Figure 3-4). Labels must be placed on each image to identify the breast quadrant and distance from the nipple.[8]

Ultrasound Guided Breast Needle Aspiration/Biopsy

Hand-held real-time imaging may be used to guide aspiration-biopsy even when the ultrasonically imaged lesion is not palpable. The lesion is first imaged and its depth and diameters are measured with electronic calipers (Figure 3-5A). Notation is made of the angle of the transducer that allows the sound wave to traverse the center of the lesion (Figure 3-5B). The transducer may be enclosed in

Figure 3-5. Cyst aspiration.

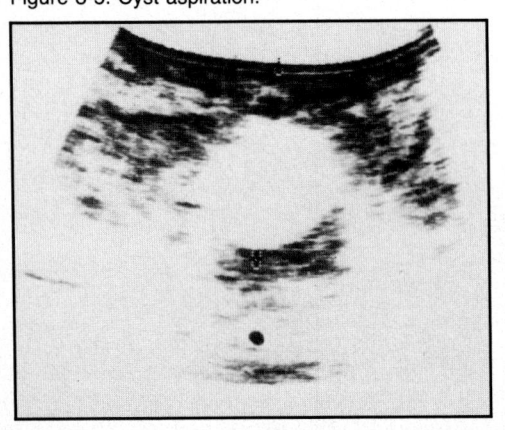

Figure 3-5A. Large 2.6cm cyst, imaged just prior to aspiration. Calipers will record depth from skin to center of cyst.

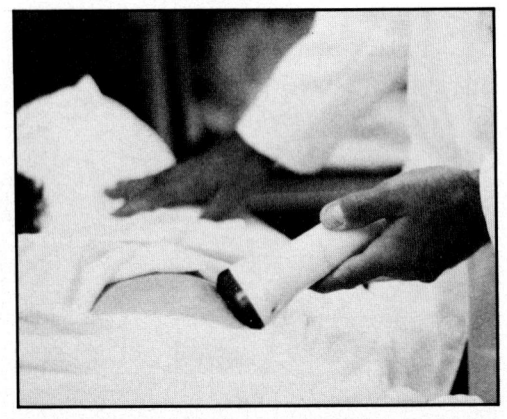

Figure 3-5B. Angle at which transducer portrays cyst at center of image.

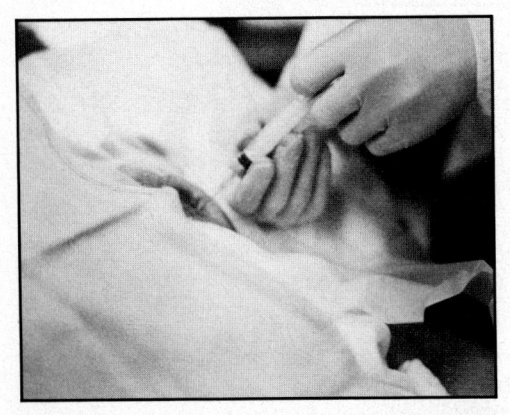

Figure 3-5C. A 20-gauge needle is inserted at same angle and to approximate depth recorded in image 3-5A.

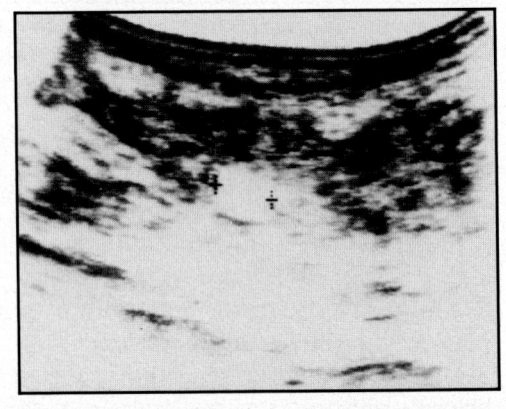

Figure 3-5D. Cyst following aspiration. Its diameter has diminished to 6mm. Aspirated fluid may be retained for cytological examination.

a sterile plastic envelope and used for needle guidance, although a 20-gauge needle is usually not sonographically visible.[9] Most physicians prefer to record the angle of the transducer and depth of the lesion instead of using the transducer during the aspiration. The biopsy site is sterilized and sterile-draped. The physician positions a 20-

gauge needle at the same angle as the transducer and marks the needle to correspond to the depth of the lesion (Figure 3-5C). The needle is inserted to that depth and an attempt is made to aspirate the lesion. After aspiration the lesion is scanned again (Figure 3-5D).

Real-Time Summary

Real-time breast imaging is fast, accurate for checking palpable lesions, and provides better resolution (at over 5MHz) than present automated scanners. Unlike long water-path automated scanners, which may not always image the edges of masses nor fully image the breast, real-time transducers can be moved around a lesion to verify its borders. However, because the field of view is limited in real-time images, the whole breast cannot be included in a single image. Hand-held transducer scanning does not produce evenly spaced planes. Finally, labelling each slice is a time consuming and tedious operation, which, if abridged or omitted by a harried sonographer, may lead to interperative confusion.

AUTOMATED INSTRUMENTS

Three automated breast scanning units are currently being commercially marketed, and images from each of these are to be found throughout this book. The word "automated" is not precise in describing these units because considerable skill and experience on the part of the technologist is required for operation, positioning, and selecting the image parameters. While the units vary in convenience, image quality, and optional imaging maneuvers, a trade-off exists between these features. Each unit, therefore, has comparative advantages and limitations when compared to the others.

Technicare

The patient lies prone with one breast at a time submerged in a water tank (Figure 3-6A). Water is chlorinated by the technologist and heated to 100°F. The breast is compressed with a plastic sheet.

50   breast ultrasound

Figure 3-6. Technicare unit.

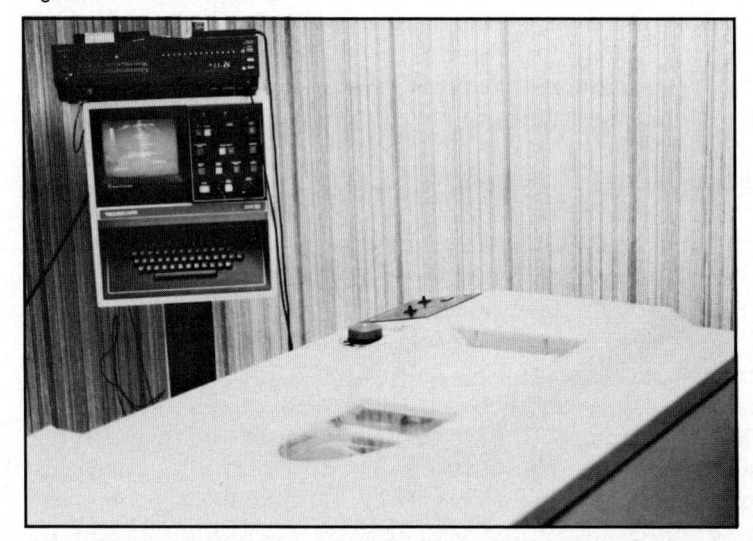

Figure 3-6A. Patient lies prone with one breast immersed in water bath.

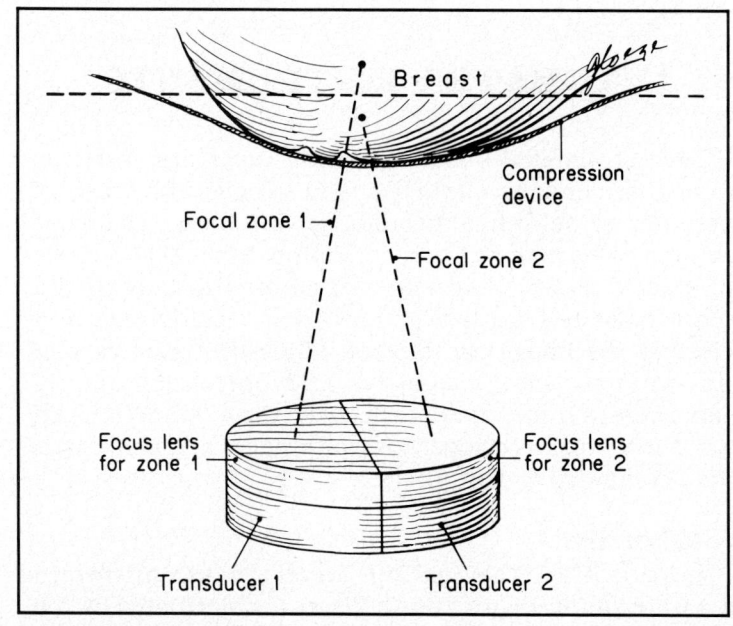

Figure 3-6B. Two transducers; each occupies half of the round cylinder and is focused at a different depth.

This unit is the easiest to operate and takes the least time for a complete examination. However, because of its inflexibility it lacks some of the diagnostic capabilites of other machines. The Technicare unit has two large-aperture 4.2MHz transducers mounted in a single fixture, so as to look like a single transducer (Figure 3-6B). Each transducer is focused at a different depth and therefore is responsible for forming only a part of the image. The two images are joined together to form an in-focus image; some image blur may occur at the boundary of the two image sections. This clever design avoids having to move the transducer assembly to bring breasts of different sizes into focus. By a sweeping motion of the transducer as the whole assembly moves across the breast, sagittal slices of 1.7mm separation are rapidly produced. However, because the transducers are not symmetrical, the slice thickness is broader than the lateral resolution. (Tests with a thread test object revealed a slice thickness of 1.2cm.) When a lesion or suspicious area is found, the unit can produce transverse slices through the area of interest. The images contain 64 gray levels. The TGC is set with three dials; when the TGC is applied, the TGC and an amplitude plot of the received signal through the breast can be visually displayed in the form of a curve.

Since a TV monitor mounted in the bottom of the water tank allows the technologist to center the nipple in the tank, positioning of the patient is an easy task. Compression of the breast is also easily performed, since the compression device is part of the scanning tank and can be tightened or loosened with a ratcheted knob. Typical examination times for both breasts are in the range of 10 to 15 minutes.

Ausonics

The Ausonics unit is similar in appearance to the Technicare (Figure 3-7A). The patient lies prone with one breast at a time submerged in the water bath. The water is heated to 98°F and chlorinated by the technologist. The breast can be compressed or allowed to hang freely during imaging, but most breasts require compression for complete penetration.

Four transducers, currently 3.9MHz or 4.5MHz, surround

52 breast ultrasound

Figure 3-7. Ausonics unit.

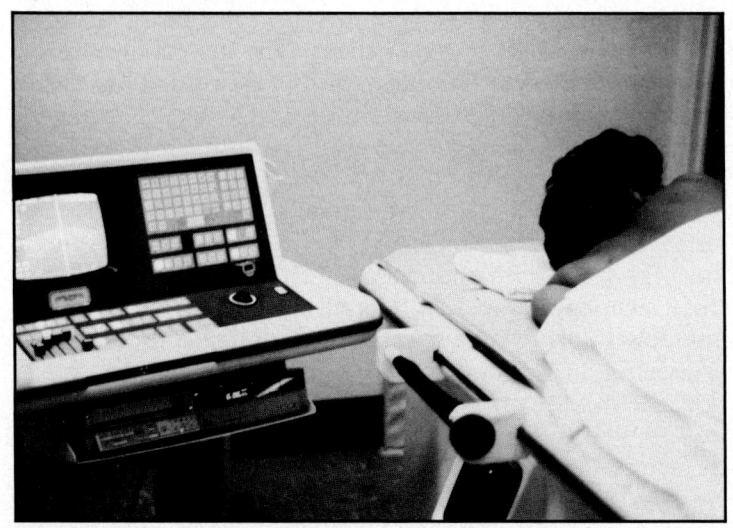

Figure 3-7A. Patient prone and slightly oblique.

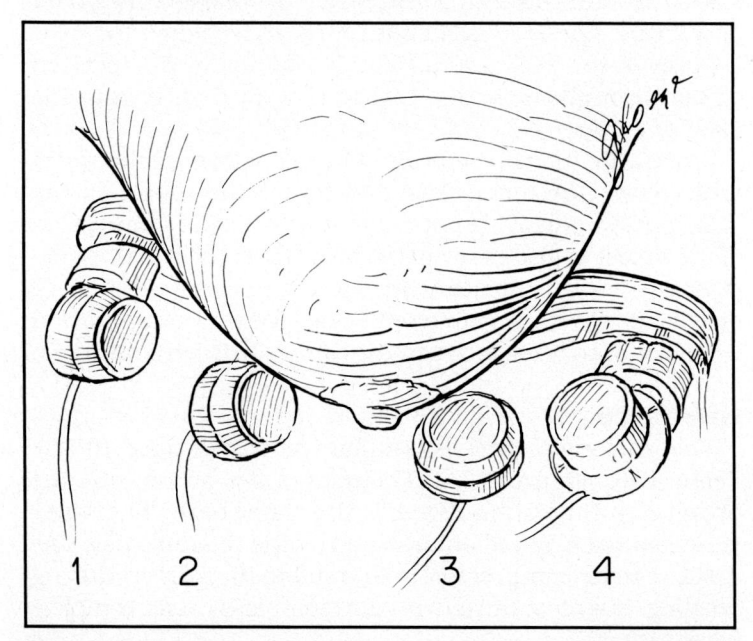

Figure 3-7B. Any combination of one to four transducers can be used to image breast.

the breast (Figure 3-7B). They are mounted in line on an arm that can rotate or move in the X or Y direction at variable step intervals. The TGC is set with sliders; the first slider is increased until the skin line can be clearly seen on the breast. This is the "trigger level" and the same TGC is applied on all subsequent echoes. The 16 gray levels can be assigned by use of several preprocessing gray level maps, but only one of these is satisfactory for breast imaging. Similarly, although several postprocessing gray level maps are offered, only one creates an acceptable image. Postprocessing reduces the number of gray levels displayed.

The arm holding the transducers can move up or down in the tank, increasing or decreasing the distance between the transducers and the breast. The technologist can position the focal zone according to the varying breast sizes and the varying depths of interest within the breast. When a suspicious area is noticed during an incremental series, it can be "remembered" by pressing a button on the console. After the series is complete, the machine can "recall" that position and return to it for additional imaging. Two, three, or four transducers can image in a compound mode or, alternatively, one or two transducers on opposite sides of the breast can be selected to scan each half of the breast, with the two images combined to form a full breast image (split screen). Compression is inconvenient if the patient is first examined with her breast uncompressed. This is because the patient must sit up while the technologist inserts a plastic window screen in the tank, following which the breast must be repositioned in the tank.

The nipple must be centered in the tank so that it can be used as a landmark for automatic labelling. Centering the nipple is accomplished by looking through a window in the tank (for gross adjustments) and then using the scanned images for the final adjustment of the positioning. Positioning both breasts twice, once free hanging and once compressed, can itself take up to five minutes of examination time.

Because of all the options available, an Ausonics bilateral examination of a symptomatic patient can take as long as 50 minutes. However, some experienced technologists can

54 breast ultrasound

Figure 3-8. Labsonics unit.

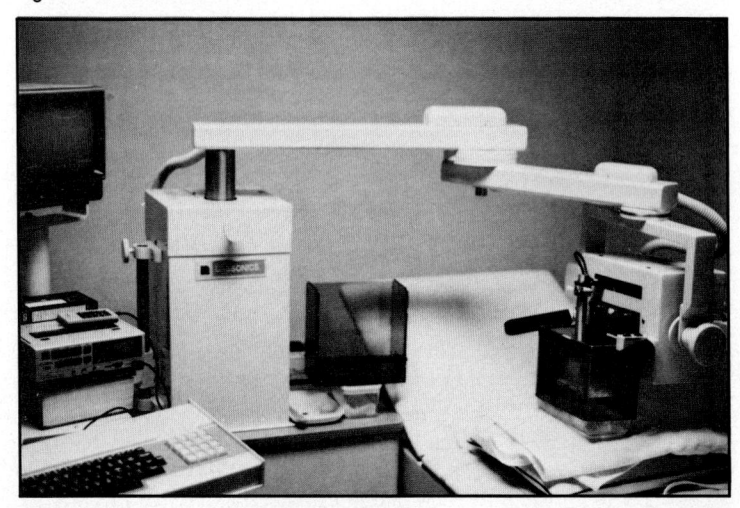

Figure 3-8A. It bears similarities to B-mode unit, except that transducer (far right) is housed in water bath.

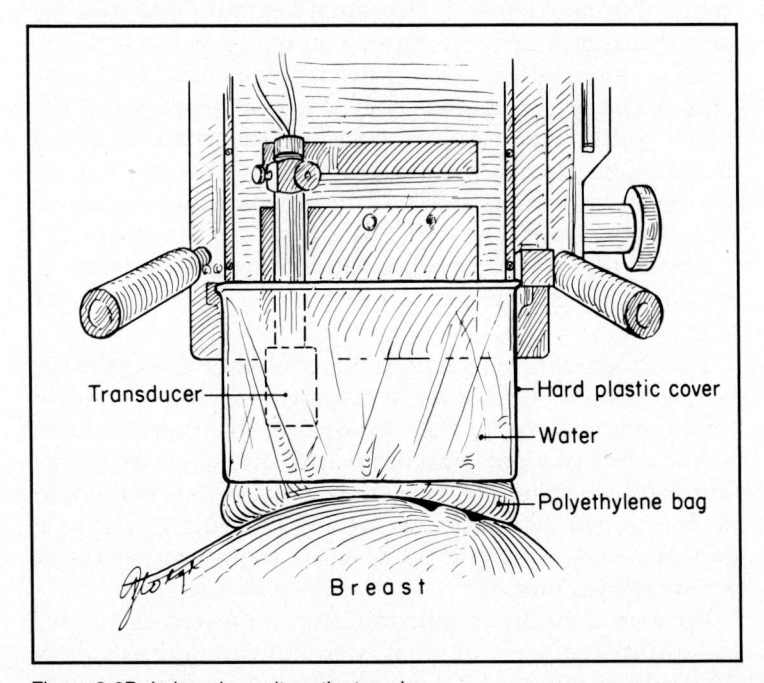

Figure 3-8B. Labsonics unit, patient supine.

complete a bilateral examination of an asymptomatic patient within 20 minutes.

Labsonics

This unit is similar to a static B-mode scanner except that the scanning arm, instead of being controlled by the technologist, is moved by a remote controlled motor in a linear pattern over the compressed breast (Figure 3-8A). The patient is supine, in the same position as for a real-time examination, so the breast is compressed by its own weight. Manipulation of the bodyposition in conjunction with angulation and compression of a polyethelene-enclosed water bath attached to the scanning arm is used to achieve the best angle of entrance of the sound beam. A sharply focused 4MHz transducer submerged in the water bag (Figure 3-8B) moves in a rectilinear pattern to form transverse, diagonal, or longitudinal slices at intervals of 1mm or greater.[10] Since the water bag can be moved to any position, the technologist can obtain oblique slices and can even image the axilla. The focal zone can be placed at any depth within the breast by use of a mechanical micrometer, which controls the vertical position of the transducer within the water bag. There is no change in compression of the breast when this technique is used. The chosen placement of the focal zone is displayed on the monitor.

The transducer moves under computer control within the water bag to form nine images. After scanning any one region or quadrant of the breast, the water bag is manually moved to the next designated region. The technologist enters the new breast quadrant data, and this information automatically appears on each breast image. Overall system gain is controlled by the sonographer in precisely calibrated dB steps. A specifically designed, non-adjustable TGC is standard, but causes some cysts deep within the breast to have less posterior enhancement than might be seen with the other units. The images are fine grained, with the appearance of good static (B-mode) scans.

The time required for a complete examination depends on the size of the breast and the number of suspicious areas, which require 1mm spaced slices. On the average,

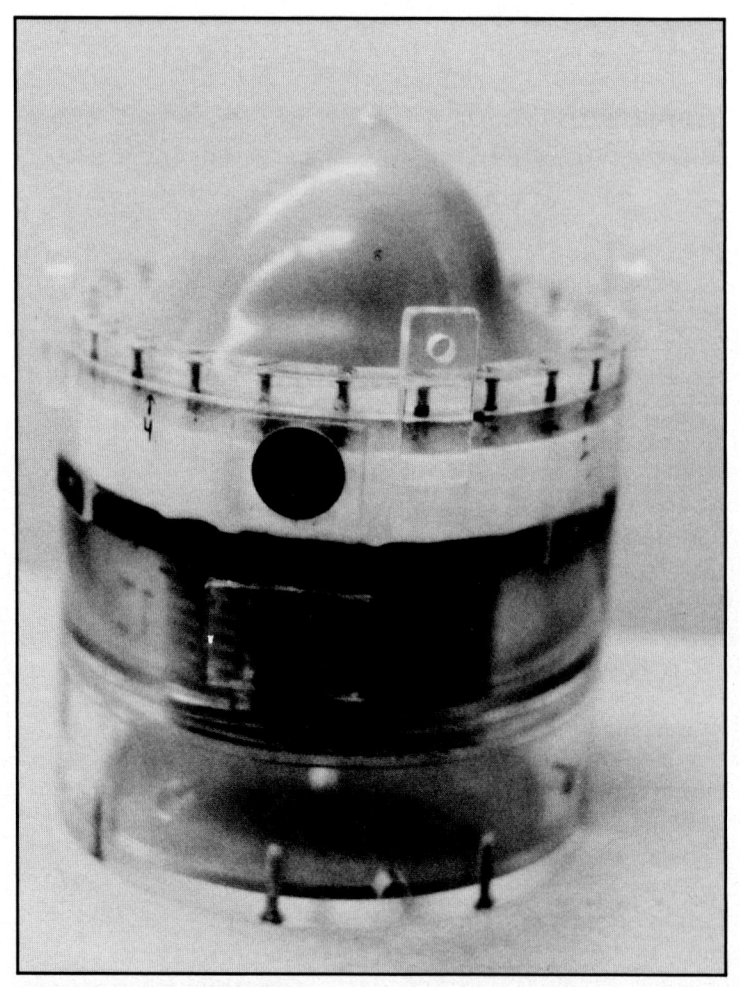

Figure 3-9. RMI breast phantom.

30 minutes are required for routine scanning of both breasts. The water in the water bag is not heated, but can be maintained at body temperature by resting the water bag on a heating pad between scans.

QUALITY CONTROL AND CALIBRATION

Real-time instruments can be checked by standard quality control procedures using either a soft scanning window test object or a thread test object submerged in a water tank.[11,12] The sponge-balloon sandwich test object described earlier can also be used to evaluate equipment performance.

Ultrasonic breast phantoms are available for both real-time and automated imaging (Figure 3-9). Although expensive, they provide realistic and accurate images that are excellent for training and for illustrating machine malfunction to a service engineer. The components of these phantoms have been carefully chosen to correspond to the acoustic properties of breast tissues,[13,14,15] and are preferred for quality control over a thread test object by some sonographers.

The Technicare and Ausonics units can be calibrated with the thread test object described in Chapter 2 (the Labsonics instrument requires a flatter test object; the built-in TGC makes quantitative calibration more difficult). If the TGC is set level to reflect the lack of attenuation in water, lateral resolution can be determined by the shape of the thread reflections in the images of the thread test object (Figure 3-10). Similarly, electronic caliper accuracy, sensitivity, and axial resolution can also be determined. Slice thickness calibration is accomplished by turning the test object 90° in the beam (Figure 3-11). These tests will help predict impending equipment failure as well as identify any failed components. Dependable imaging requires careful matching of the sensitivities of the two Technicare and the four Ausonics transducers.

References

1. Ophir J, Maklad NF: Digital scan converters in diagnostic ultrasound imaging. Proc IEEE 67:654-664, 1979.
2. Maklad NF, Johnson M, Bowie JD, et al: Diagnostic ultrasound imaging. Invest Radiol 19:58-12, 1984.
3. Thickman DI, Ziskin MC, Goldenberg NJ: Effect of display format on detectability. J Ultrasound Med 2:117-122, 1983.

58 breast ultrasound

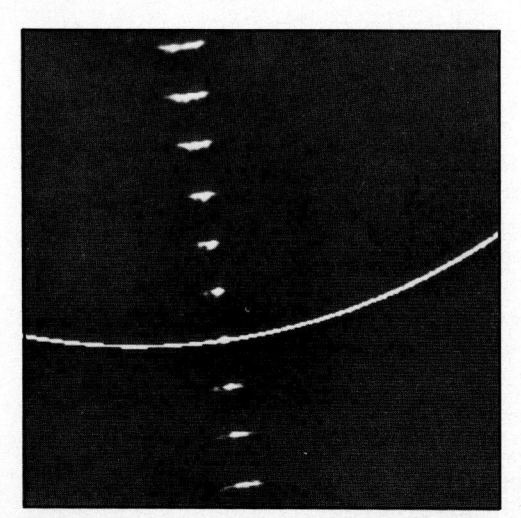

Figure 3-10. Lateral resolution. Thread test object from Figure 3-2, flat TGC. Arc indicates focal zone. Top three lines represent distorted cross-sections of threads in near field. Next four cross-section images of threads are sharper since they are closer to focal zone.

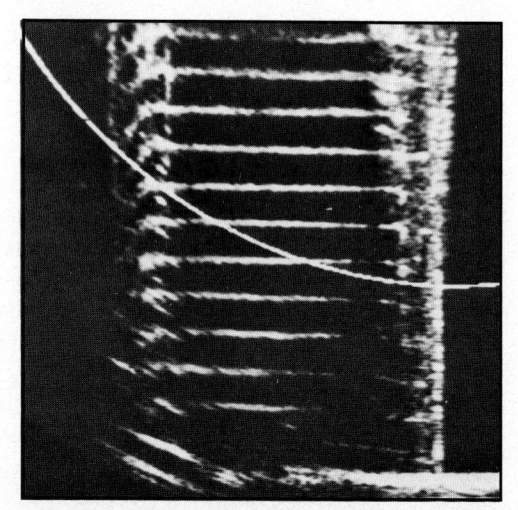

Figure 3-11. Slice thickness. Thread test object, rotated 90°. Arc indicates focal zone. Slice thickness is measured as transducer moves away from test object. Slice thickness represents distance transducer can move and still image test object.

4. Robinson DE, Knight PC: Interpolation scan conversion in pulse-echo ultrasound. Ultrasonic Imaging 4:297-310, 1982.

5. King W, Kimme-Smith C, Winter J: Renal stone shadowing: an investigation of contributing factors. Radiology 154:191-196, 1985.

6. Winter J, Kimme-Smith C, King W: Measurement accuracy of sonographic sector scanners. AJR 144:645-648, 1985.

7. Goldstein A, Madrazo BL: Slice-thickness artifacts in gray-scale ultrasound. JCU 9:365-376, 1981.

8. Baum G: Labeling of meridional and radiol scans of the breast. J Ultrasound Med 2:363-368, 1983.

9. Heckeman R, Seidel KJ: The sonographic appearance and contrast enhancement of puncture needles. JCU 11:265-268, 1983.

10. Kelly-Fry, Harper AP: Factors critical to highly accurate diagnosis of matched breast pathologies by ultrasound imaging. *In* Lerski RA, Morley P (eds): Ultrasound '82. New York: Permagon Press, 1983, p 415.

11. Benjavic RA: Design and maintenance of a quality control assurance program for diagnostic ultrasound equipment. Seminars in Ultrasound 4:10, 1983.

12. Goldstein A: Quality Assurance in Diagnostic Ultrasound. U.S. Department of Health and Human Services, HHS Publication 81-8139.

13. Madsen EL, Zagzebski JA, Banjavic RA, et al: Tissue mimicking materials for ultrasound phantoms. Med Phys 5:391-394, 1978.

14. Madsen EL, Zagzebski JA, Frank GR, et al: Anthropomorphic breast phantoms for assessing ultrasonic imaging system performance and for training ultrasonographers: Part I. J Clin Ultrasound 10:67-75, 1982.

15. Madsen EL, Zagzebski JA, Frank GR: An anthropomorphic ultrasound breast phantom containing intermediate-sized scatterers. Ultrasound in Med and Biol 3:381-392, 1982.

CHAPTER 4

The Normal Breast

INTRODUCTION

The breast is composed of fat, lactiferous ducts and lobules (collectively called the parenchyma), and connective tissue. Because the amount of each of these tissues greatly varies not only with age and parity, but also among women of the same age and parity, it is impossible for a single ultrasound image to be considered representative of all normal breasts. Therefore, this chapter will contain a variety of sonograms of the normal breasts of women who differ in age and parity. Many of these normal ultrasound images will be correlated with their x-ray mammographic counterparts.

ANATOMY

The breast can conveniently be divided into four distinct anatomical regions: 1) the region comprising the skin, nipple and subareolar structures, 2) the subcutaneous region, 3) the parenchymal region, and 4) the retromammary region (Figure 4-1).[1] The subcutaneous region is composed of fat lobules and distal extensions of the suspensory ligaments of Cooper. These ligaments are connective tissue septa that enclose parenchymal lobules throughout the breast, extending from the juxtathoracic deep layer of superficial fascia to the skin. The cone-shaped parenchymal region includes the functional elements (mammary lobules and ducts), connective tissue, suspensory ligaments, and varying amounts of fat. The retromammary region, a thin layer of fat, separates the parenchyma from the fascia overlying the pectoralis muscles.

ULTRASOUND OF THE NORMAL BREAST

The breast is composed of fatty, parenchymal (ducts and lobules), and connective tissues. Of these, the acoustic

Figure 4-1. Breast anatomy.

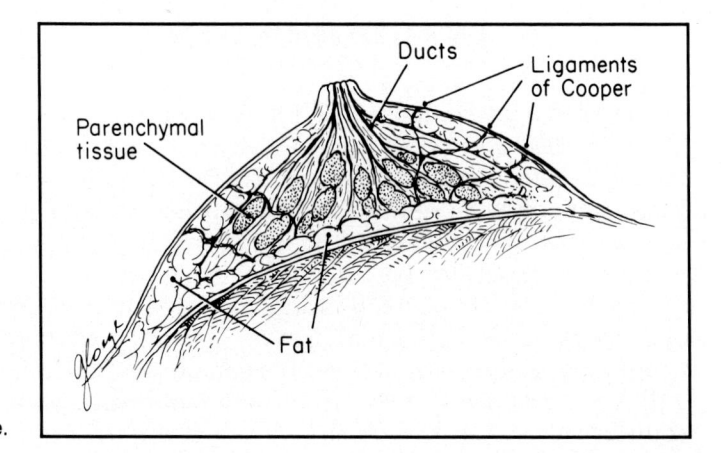

Figure 4-1A. Transverse plane.

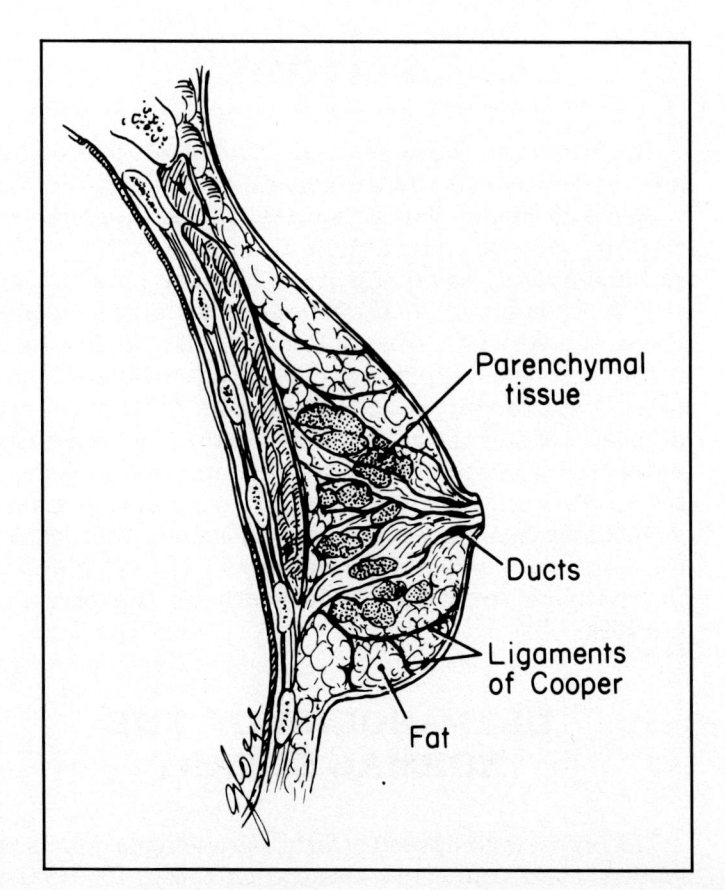

Figure 4-1B. Sagittal plane.

the normal breast **65**

Figure 4-2. Normal breast ultrasound, bilaterally symmetrical, 54-year-old woman. S = subcutaneous fat; P = parenchymal layer; M = pectoralis muscle; L = ligaments of Cooper; R = rib.

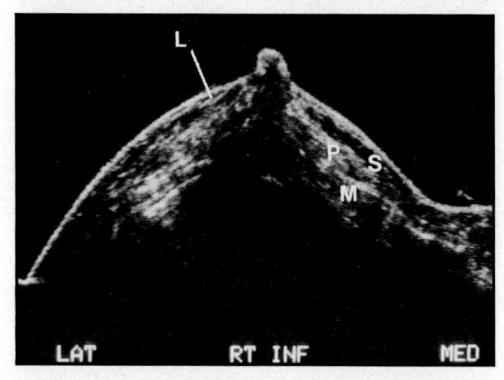

Figure 4-2A,B. Transverse whole breast image of non-compressed, free-hanging right (A) and left (B) breasts. Note bilateral symmetry. Deeper tissue is not penetrated because of insufficient power.

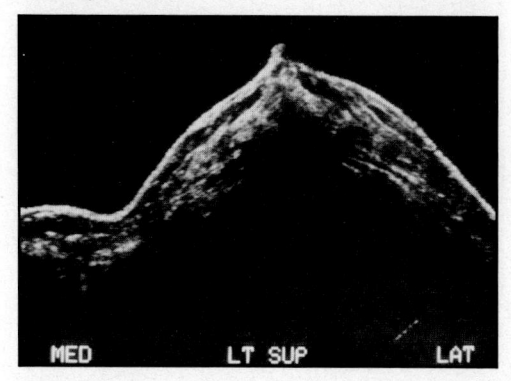

Figure 4-2B.

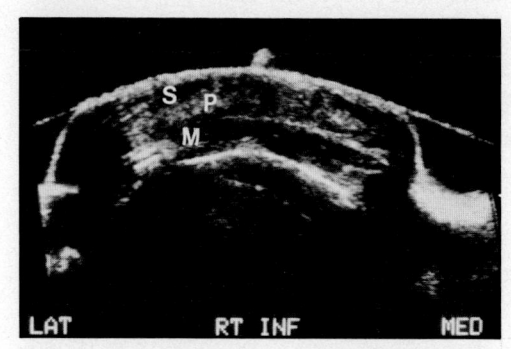

Figure 4-2C,D. Transverse whole breast images of compressed right (C) and left (D) breasts. With compression, deeper tissue is adequately penetrated, but lateral aspect is poorly penetrated because of critical angle refraction off skin and fat/parenchymal interface.

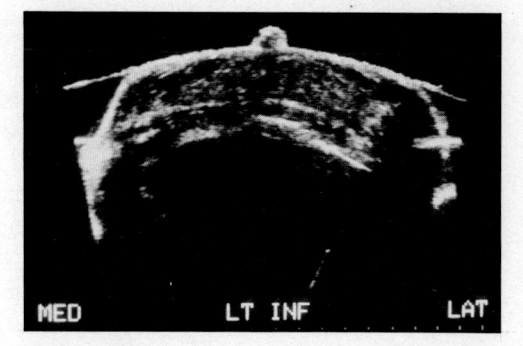

Figure 4-2D.

impedance of fat is lowest, that of parenchymal tissue is intermediate, and that of connective tissue is highest. Dense connective tissue manifests greater acoustic attenuation than loose connective tissue. These differences in attenuation of the ultrasound beam are an important factor

66 breast ultrasound

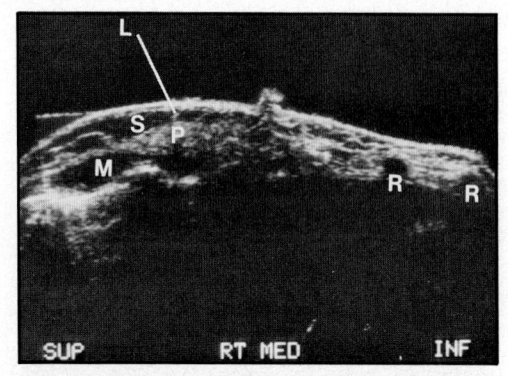

Figure 4-2E,F. Sagittal whole breast images of compressed right (E) and left (F) breasts. (Ausonics)

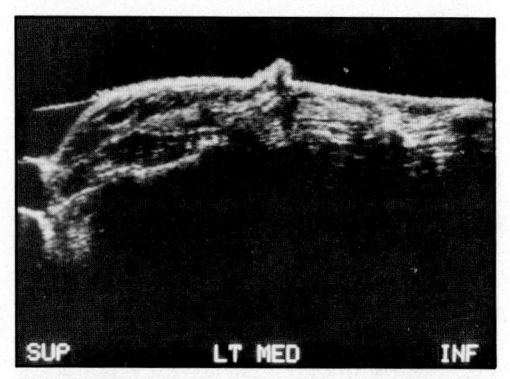

Figure 4-2F.

in the production of the sonomammographic image. Normal breasts tend to be bilaterally symmetrical in their echographic appearance (Figure 4-2).[2] Asymmetry in the echoic pattern may be the only sign of pathology.

Region of the Skin, Nipple and Subareolar Structures

Normal skin appears as a thin, uniform, highly reflective line 0.5mm to 2mm thick. Thickened skin is characterized by a widened specular reflection. In water-path scanning, thickened skin may result in a bright specular epidermal reflection at the water-skin interface.[3]

The nipple contains a large amount of connective tissue that, in combination with the dense connective tissue surrounding the subareolar ducts, can lead to acoustic shadowing sufficiently prominent to prevent the visualization of an underlying mass (Figure 4-3). Reflection and refraction from the obliquely oriented sides of the protruding nipple contribute to the shadowing. Caution must be exerted to guard against misinterpreting this shadow as a subareolar cancer.[4] The extent of the shadowing may be reduced by applying sufficient compression that the nipple does not protrude beyond the contour of the breast surface. In addition, compound scanning with multidirectional transducers may obliterate the shadow.

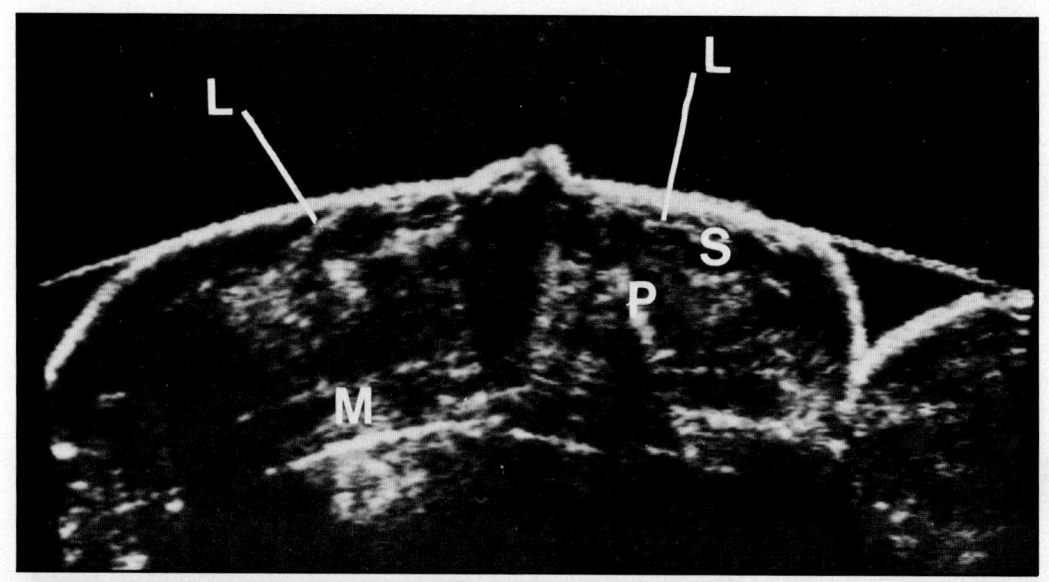

Figure 4-3. Nipple shadowing. The nipple casts an acoustic shadow to the chest wall; compressed breast of a 45-year-old woman. L = ligaments of Cooper; S = subcutaneous fat; P = parenchymal tissue; M = pectoral muscle.

Although the deeper segments of the lactiferous ducts are usually collapsed, they cast narrow cylindrical shadows secondary to the acoustic attenuation of the surrounding dense connective tissue. In contrast, the subareolar ampullary segments are normally dilated, and can be identified as sonolucent tubular structures 2mm to 8mm in diameter (Figure 4-4). Generalized ductal dilatation is characteristic of the lactating breast.

Subcutaneous Region

Since echo amplitudes at tissue interfaces are a function of the differences in their acoustic impedance, the interface between the skin and subcutaneous fat and the interface between the subcutaneous fat and dense parenchymal connective tissue are readily visualized (Figure 4-2). The amplitude of the echoes at these and other interfaces is also affected by the incident angle of the ultrasound beam, being brightest where the angle is 90°. The subcutaneous region displays fine, weakly echogenic reflections from fat lobules, interspersed with strong echoes from the

68 breast ultrasound

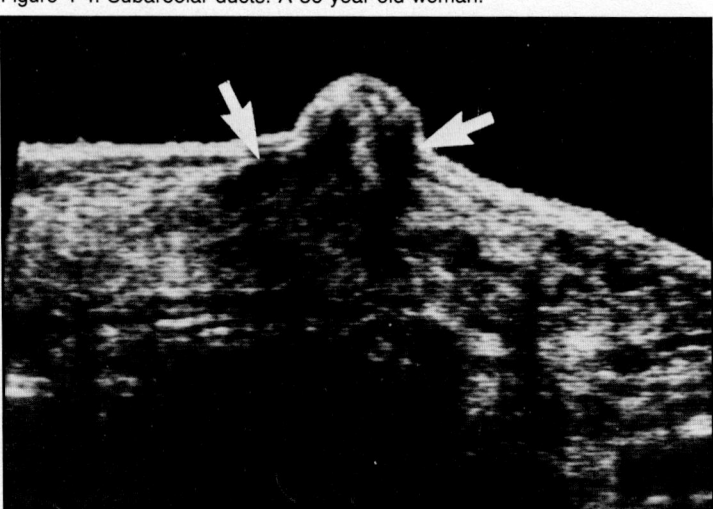

Figure 4-4. Subareolar ducts. A 36-year-old woman.

Figure 4-4A. Dedicated examination. (Ausonics)

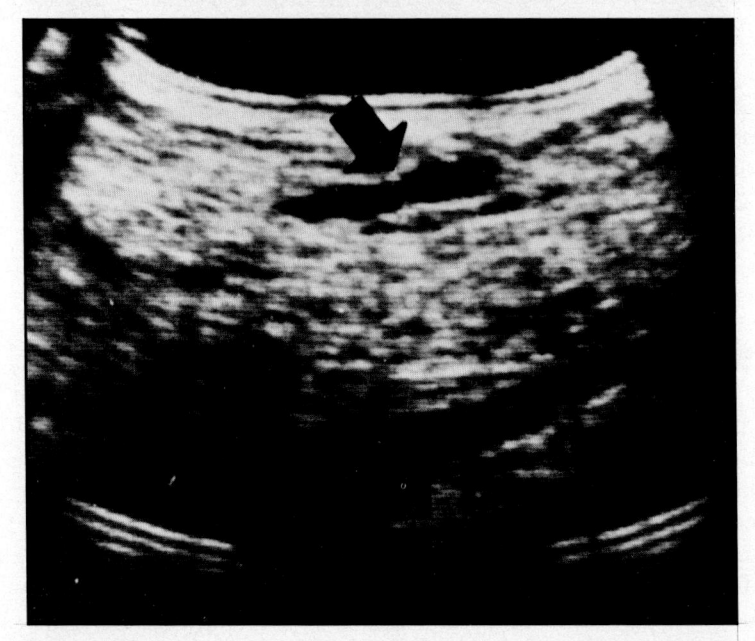

Figure 4-4B. Hand-held real-time examination shows dilated subareolar duct leading to nipple.

the normal breast 69

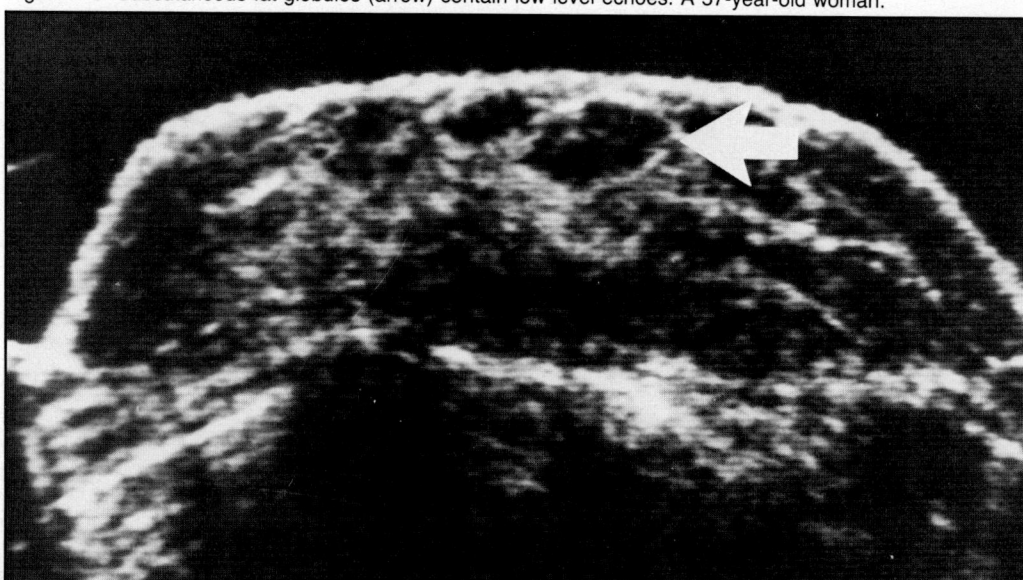

Figure 4-5. Subcutaneous fat globules (arrow) contain low level echoes. A 57-year-old woman.

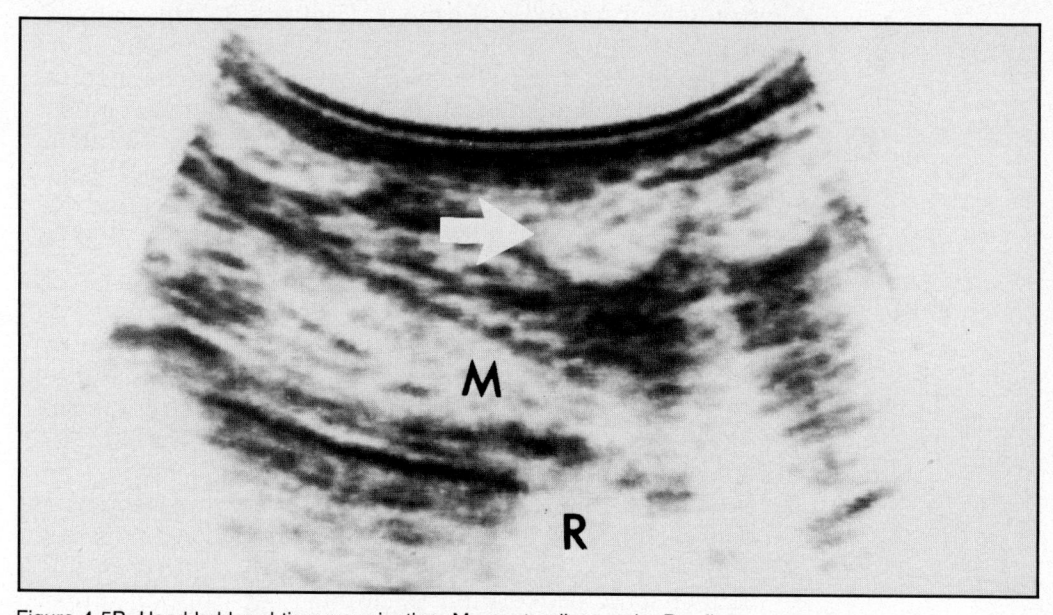

Figure 4-5A. Transverse section whole-breast examination with compression. (Ausonics)

Figure 4-5B. Hand-held real-time examination. M = pectoralis muscle; R = rib.

suspensory ligaments of Cooper (Figure 4-5). These ligaments may cast worrisome shadows when the angle of incidence of the ultrasound beam is such that considerable sound wave refraction occurs (Figure 4-6A). However, the shadows frequently disappear when the ligaments are flattened and made more perpendicular to the incident beam by breast compression (Figure 4-6B).

Mammary Parenchymal Region

The parenchyma assumes a triangular configuraton between the subcutaneous and retromammary regions. Because its sonographic appearance varies according to the relative amounts of fat and connective tissue within it, specific parenchymal ultrasound patterns may be identified. These patterns have been correlated with the x-ray mammographic parenchymal patterns described by Wolfe.[5,6,7]

Fatty Pattern. In the fatty breast, sonolucent fat lobules have replaced nearly all of the parenchymal tissue, resulting in a relatively anechoic, loose, lace-like ultrasonic appearance throughout the breast (Figure 4-7). This pattern is more frequent in older women and in women who have had many children. The fatty breast is not well-suited to ultrasound examination since the clumps of fat reflect much of the ultrasound energy and fat lobules may simulate breast masses. Moreover, a round mass surrounded by fat lobules of similar echogenicity may not be detectable. X-ray mammography, however, is highly accurate in this type of breast.

Dense Glandular or Fibrous Pattern. In this type of breast, the parenchymal region is filled with dense homogeneous connective tissue that produces strong coalescent echoes similar in intensity to those of the skin. In breasts manifesting extremely dense parenchyma, the subcutaneous fat usually consists of a very thin layer, and no fat lobules are visible within the parenchyma (Figures 4-8 and 4-9). Compression is frequently required for adequate sonic penetration by automated scanning units.

the normal breast **71**

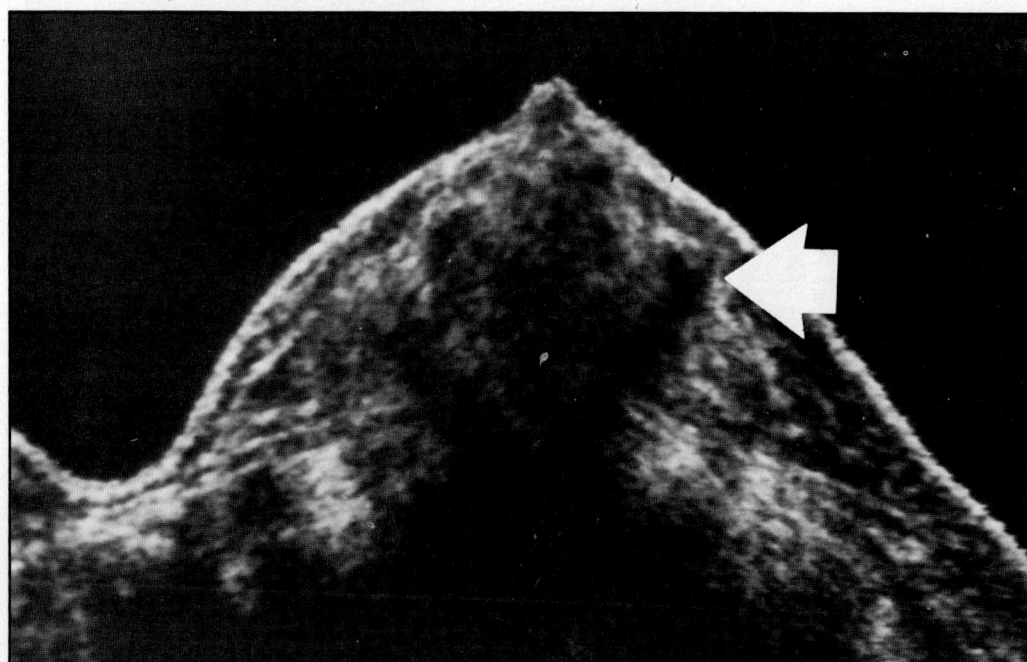

Figure 4-6. A 43-year-old woman with dense breasts on x-ray mammography.

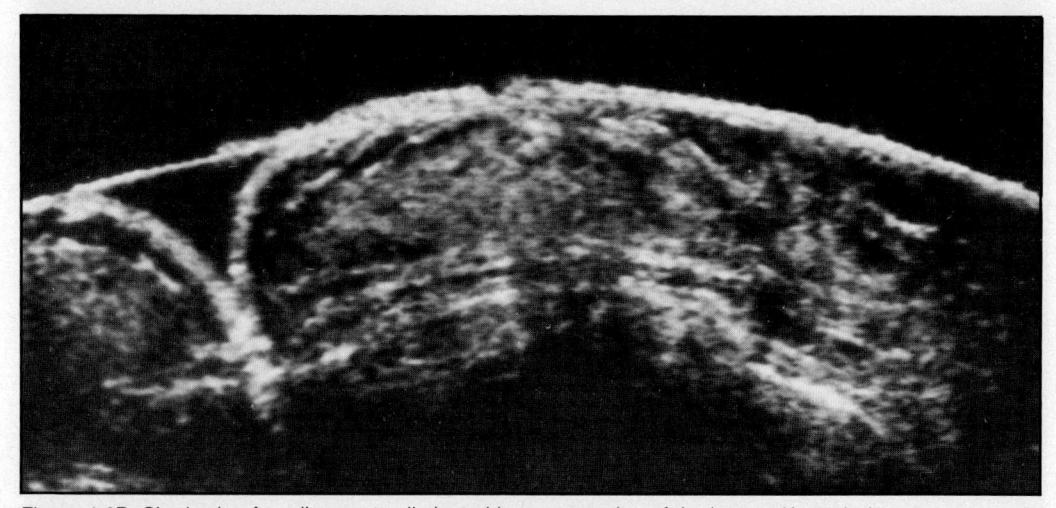

Figure 4-6A. Shadowing from refraction of sound waves at Cooper ligaments (arrow).

Figure 4-6B. Shadowing from ligaments eliminated by compression of the breast. (Ausonics)

72   breast ultrasound

Figure 4-7. Fatty breast of a 60-year-old woman.

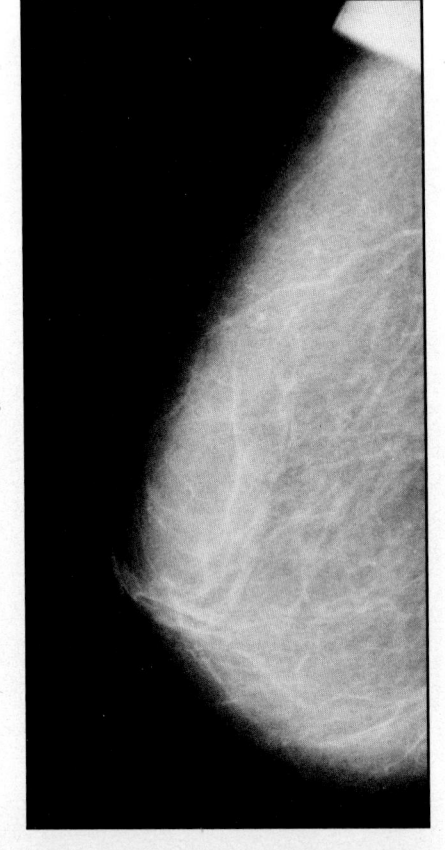

Figure 4-7A. Mediolateral film-screen mammogram shows almost complete fat replacement of parenchymal tissue.

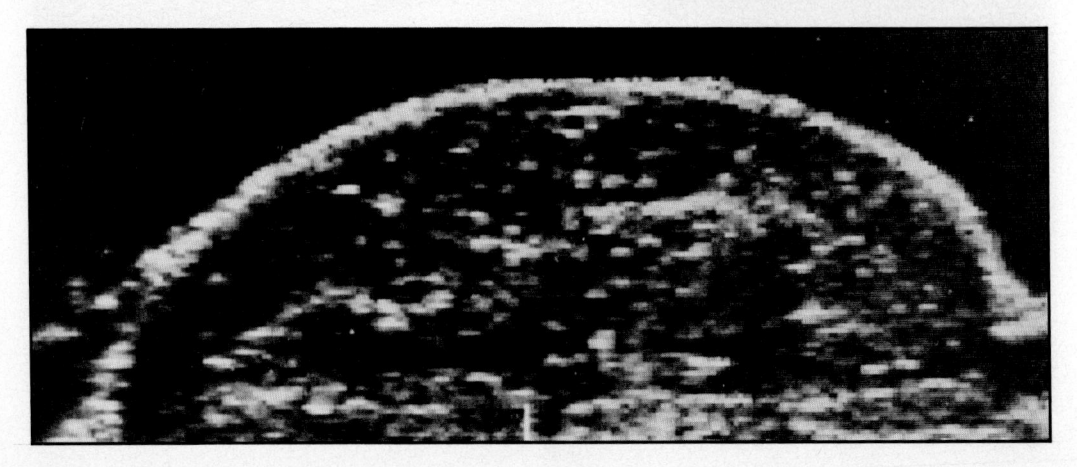

Figure 4-7B. Ultrasound. Relatively even hypoechoic echoes throughout. (Technicare)

the normal breast 73

Figure 4-8. Dense glandular pattern in a 30-year-old woman.

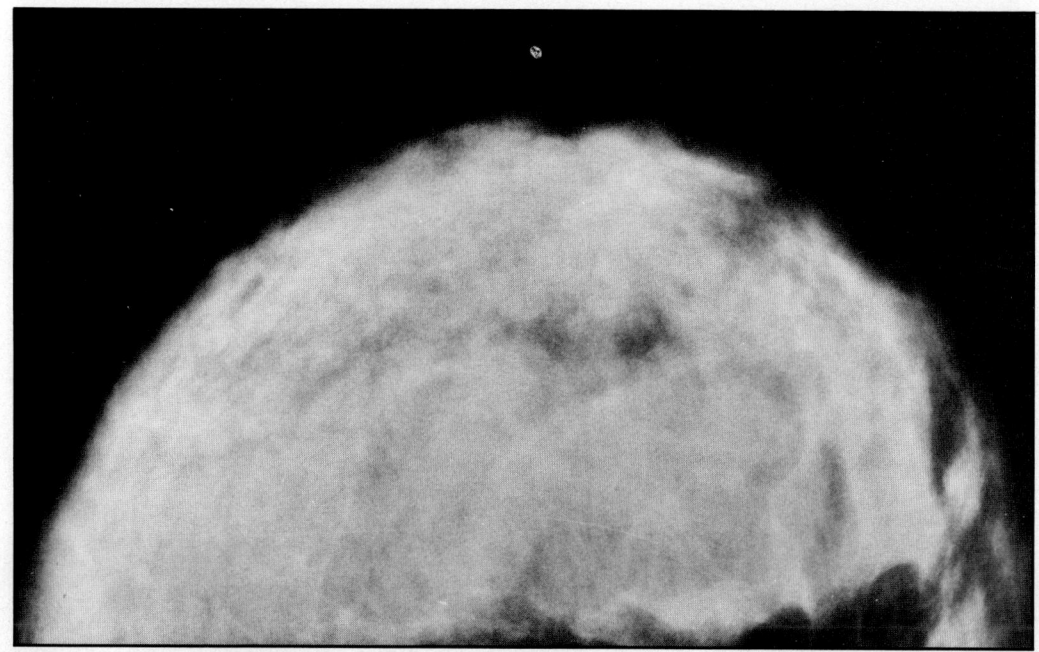

Figure 4-8A. Cephalocaudal screen-film mammograms.

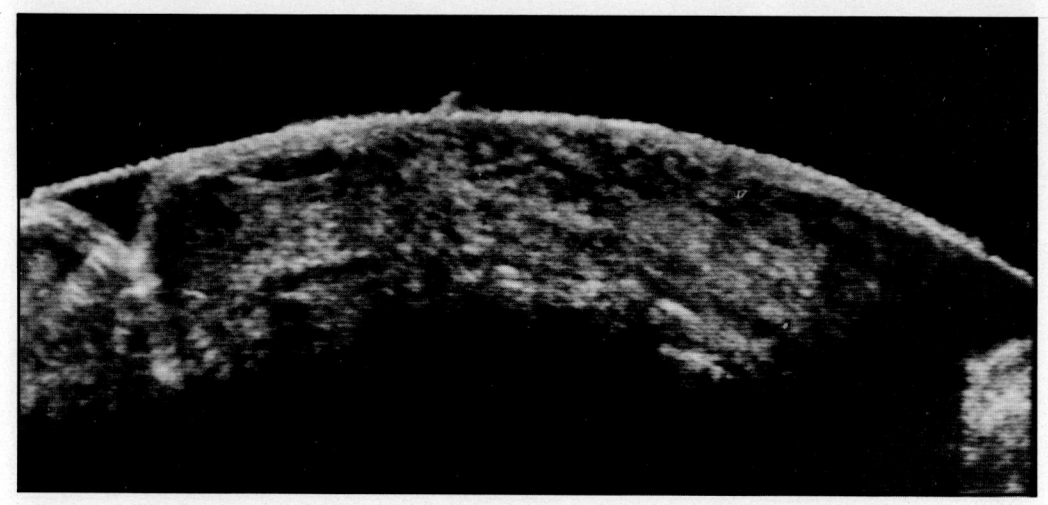

Figure 4-8B. Whole-breast ultrasound (compressed). Strong echoes throughout parenchyma (compare to skin echoes). (Ausonics)

74 breast ultrasound

Figure 4-9. A 43-year-old woman with dense parenchyma centrally.

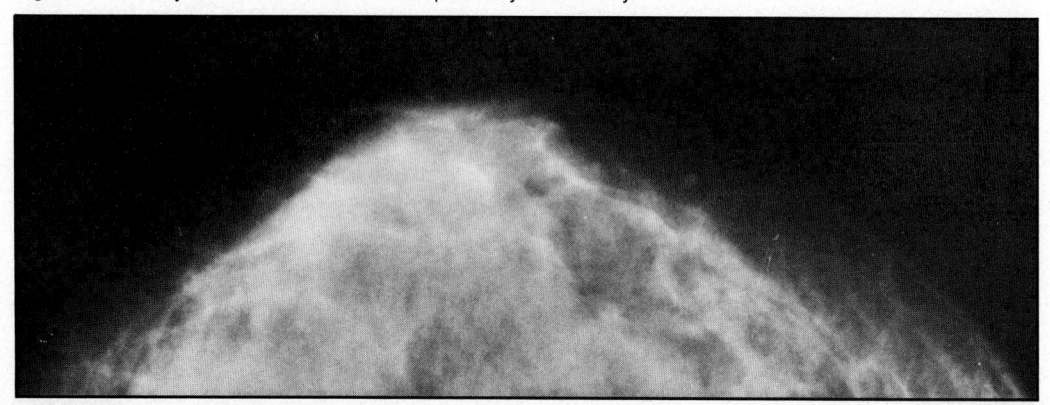

Figure 4-9A. Cephalocaudal mammogram.

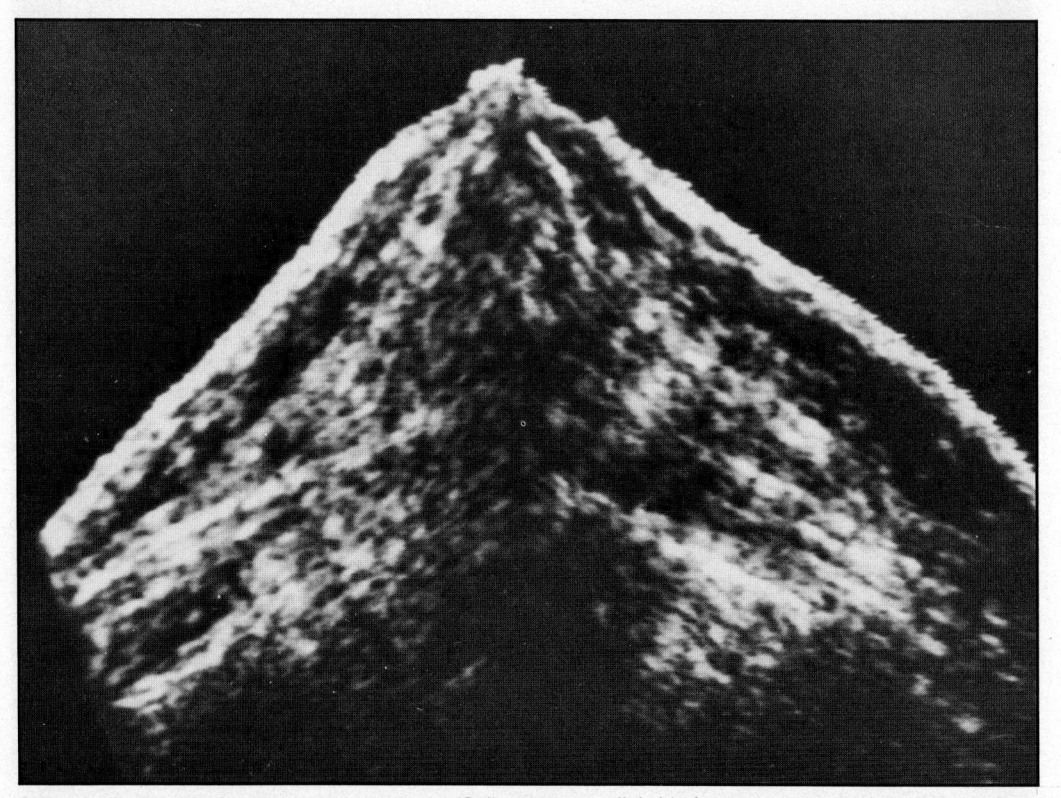

Figure 4-9B. Transverse section through nipple. (Split-screen: medial side from one transducer; lateral side from opposing transducer). (Ausonics)

Even so, attenuation of the ultrasound beam may be so severe that the deeper portions of the breast cannot be depicted even with vigorous compression and high power settings.

Mixed Fatty and Fibrous Pattern. With advancing age and child bearing, the dense glandular tissue of the parenchyma involutes and is replaced by fat (Figure 4-10). In a breast composed of a mixture of dense parenchymal tissue and fat, it is often difficult to distinguish a focus of fat replacement from a breast mass. The importance of correlating the x-ray and ultrasound mammograms to avoid pitfalls such as this cannot be overemphasized.

Prominent Ductal Pattern. Breasts with a prominent ductal pattern (periductal fibrosis, collagenosis) in x-ray mammograms may contain varying amounts of fat and dense connective tissue. In our sonographic experience, it has been the amount of fat relative to the amount of connective tissue, and not the prominence of the ducts, that has primarily determined of the appearance of the ultrasound image. Superimposed on the resultant pattern, the dense periductal connective tissue when surrounded by fat gives rise to discrete circumscribed or linear foci of echoes, slightly less in amplitude than those of the skin (Figure 4-11).

Retromammary Region

Depiction of the retromammary region ensures that there has been adequate sonographic penetration of the breast. The layer of fat in the retromammary region is thinner than in the subcutaneous region, and the fat lobules tend to be smaller. The pectoralis major muscle lies deep to the breast (Figure 4-2). The strongly echoic interface between the retromammary fat and the fascial connective tissue overlying the muscle is easily recognized. The underlying ribs cast strong acoustic shadows in sagittal sections.

76　breast ultrasound

Figure 4-10. A 48-year-old woman. Mixed fatty and fibrous pattern.

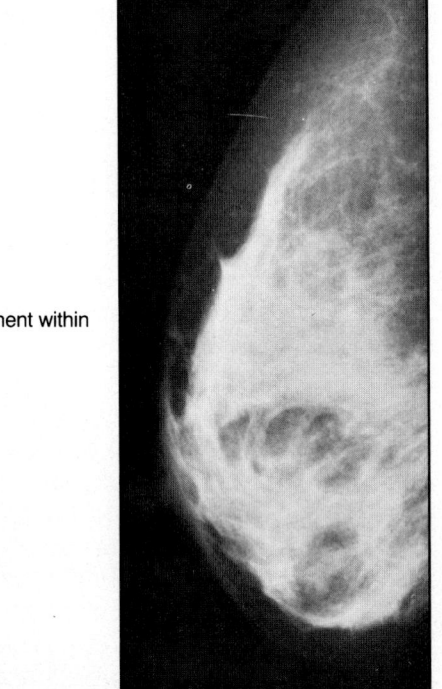

Figure 4-10A. Mediolateral mammogram shows fat replacement within dense parenchyma.

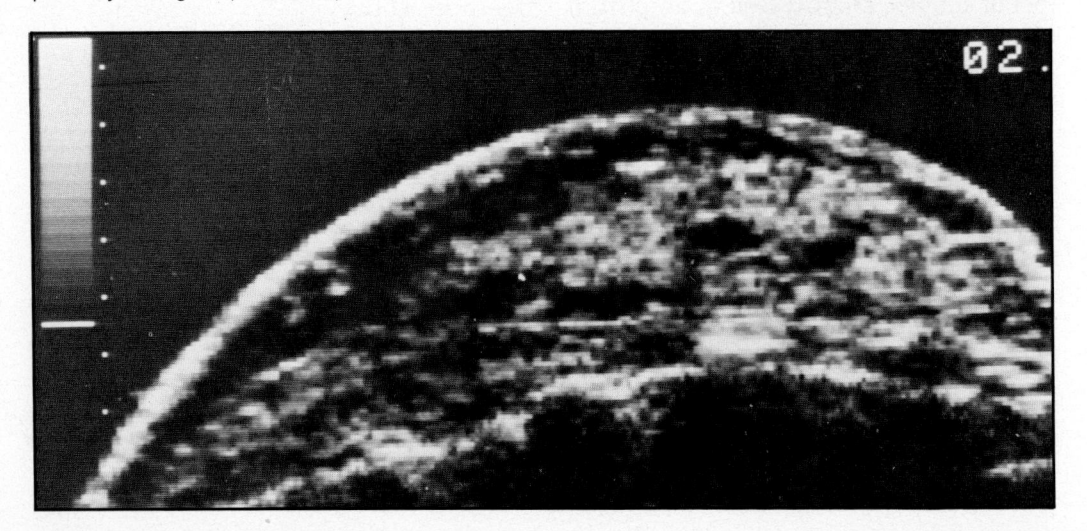

Figure 4-10B. Sagittal whole-breast section shows islands of fat within parenchymal region. (Technicare)

the normal breast **77**

Figure 4-11. Periductal fibrosis and dysplastic patterns in a 61-year-old woman. Courtesy of Wende W. Logan, MD, Buffalo, New York.

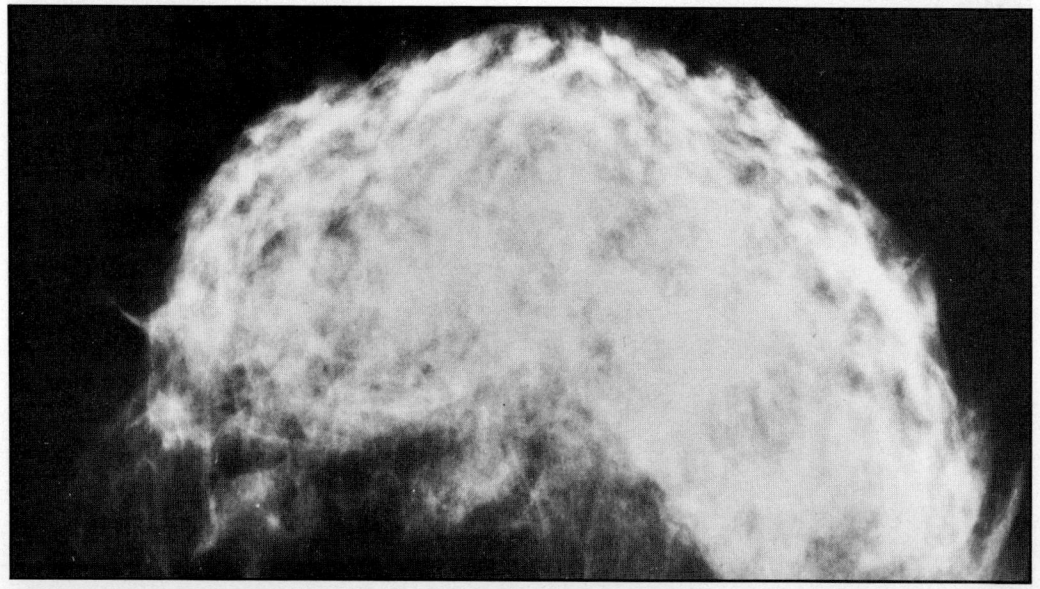

Figure 4-11A. Cephalocaudal mammogram shows mixture of discrete prominent ducts and homogeneous density.

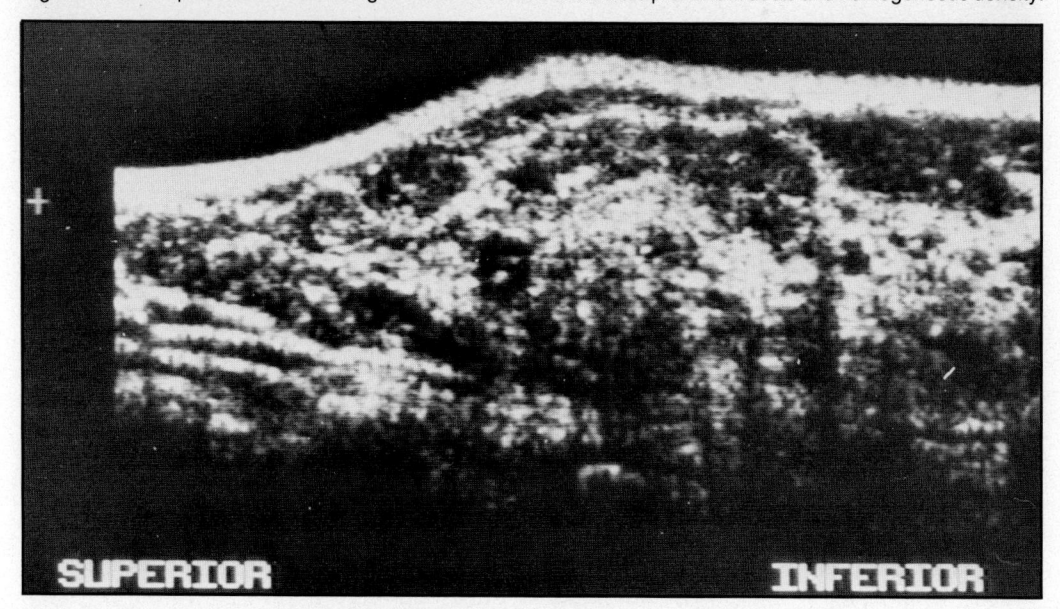

Figure 4-11B. Dedicated ultrasound, sagittal section. (Labsonics)

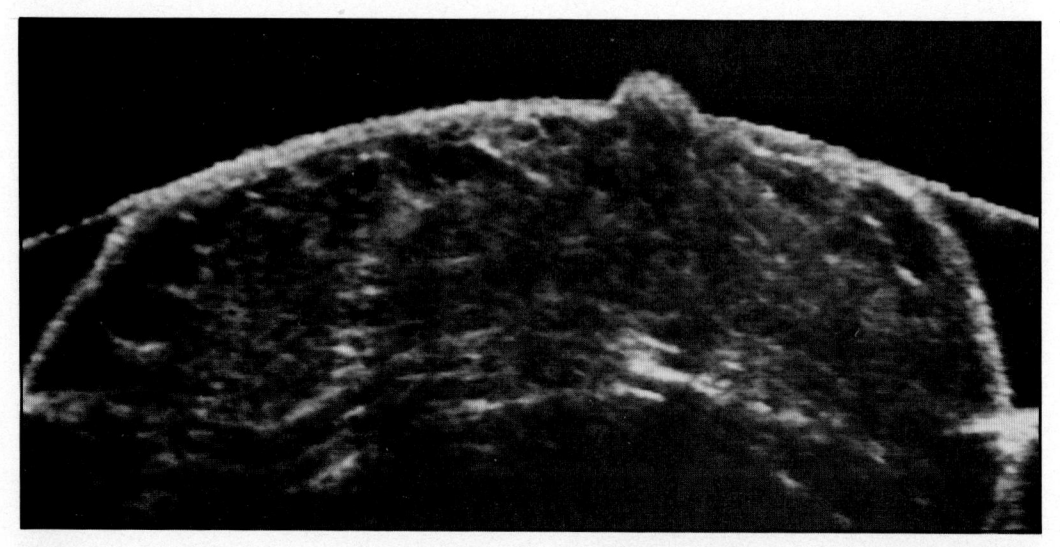

Figure 4-12. Pregnancy, in a 28-year-old. Transverse section with compression. Thin subcutaneous and retromammary regions. "Snowy," weak, uniform echoes throughout. (Ausonics)

THE PREGNANT BREAST

During pregnancy the breast undergoes proliferation of the ducts and lobules constituting the parenchyma. The proliferative process displaces and thins the subcutaneous and retromammary fat. The parenchyma manifests a "snowy" appearance characterized by weak, poorly defined, uniform echoes attributable to relatively small differences in acoustic impedance at tissue interfaces (Figure 4-12).[1]

References

1. Schneck CD, Lehman DA: Sonographic anatomy of the breast. Seminars in Ultrasound 3:13-33, 1982.
2. Kossoff G, Jellins J, Reeve TS: Ultrasound in the detection of early breast cancer, In Grundmann E (ed): Early Diagnosis of Breast Cancer. New York: Gustav Fischer Verlag, 1978, p 149.
3. Kopans DB, Meyer JE, Proppe KH: The double line of skin thickening on sonograms of the breast. Radiology 141:485-487, 1981.
4. Kobayashi T: Ultrasonic detection of breast cancer. Clin Obstet Gynecol 25:409-423, 1982.

5. Wolfe JN: Breast patterns as an index of risk for developing breast cancer. AJR 126:1130-1139, 1976.

6. Rubin CS, Kurtz AB, Goldberg BB, et al: Ultrasonic mammographic parenchymal patterns: a preliminary report. Radiology 130:515-517, 1979.

7. Cole-Beuglet C: Ultrasound, *In* Bassett LW, Gold RH (eds): Mammography, Thermography, and Ultrasound in Breast Cancer Detection. New York: Grune & Stratton, 1982, p 151.

CHAPTER 5

Benign Disorders

INTRODUCTION

Of all breast lesions, benign and malignant, ultrasound diagnosis is most sensitive and specific for cysts; cysts can be accurately identified, localized and measured by ultrasound. Fibroadenoma is a solid lesion that manifests characteristic but not pathognomonic ultrasound features; certain well-circumscribed malignancies may have sonographic features identical to those of fibroadenoma. Included in this chapter are examples of these and of cystosarcoma phylloides (usually benign, only rarely metastasizing), papilloma, lipoma, abscess, hematoma, galactocele, sebaceous cyst, and breast augmentation mammoplasty.

CYSTS

Cysts, the most frequent mass lesions of the breast in women 35 to 50 years of age, are believed to develop from the dilatation of terminal ducts.[1] The fluid-filled masses may be solitary or multiple, unilateral or bilateral. While in some patients cysts are painful and tender, in others they may go unrecognized until the patient or her physician discovers a palpable lump. Cysts may sometimes undergo a very rapid increase or decrease in size. Ultrasound is the most reliable noninvasive method for the detection of cysts including those as small as 3mm in diameter. Sonography has been reported to be 98% accurate in this endeavor.[2] Cysts are characterized by the following sonographic features: well-circumscribed margins including a definite posterior wall, round or oval contour, absence of internal echoes, and enhanced posterior echoes (Figures 5-1 through 5-7).[2-6]

84 breast ultrasound

Figure 5-1. Characteristic cysts. A 45-year-old woman felt painful lump in outer portion of left breast.

Figure 5-1A. Mediolateral mammogram shows mixed pattern with several mass densities. Exact borders of masses are obscured by surrounding fibroglandular tissue.

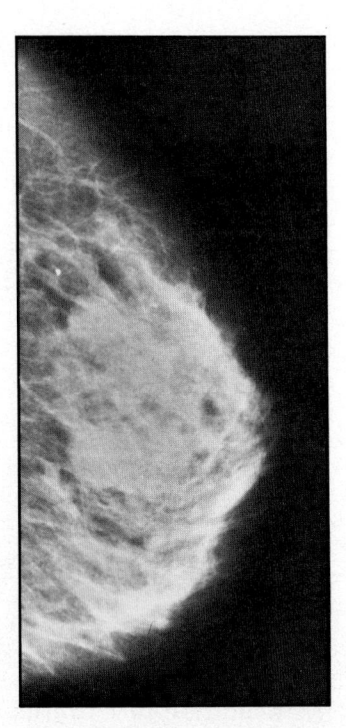

Figure 5-1B. Hand-held real-time ultrasound. Two cysts are depicted. Characteristic features are well-circumscribed margins, oval contours, absence of internal echoes, and enhanced posterior echoes, as well as enhanced surrounding parenchymal echoes due to compression by cysts.

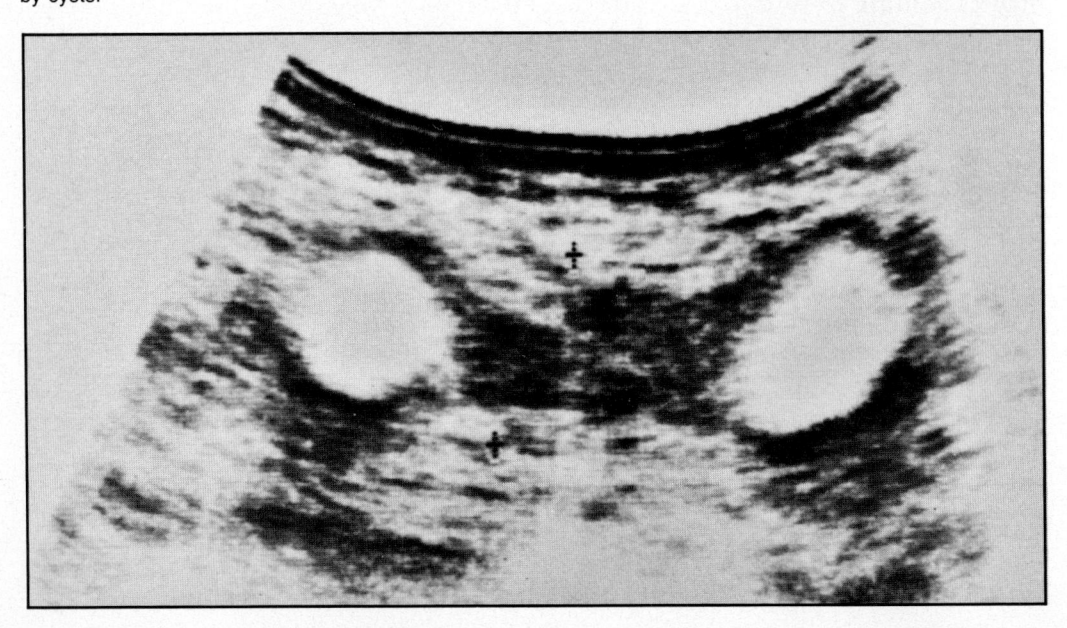

benign disorders **85**

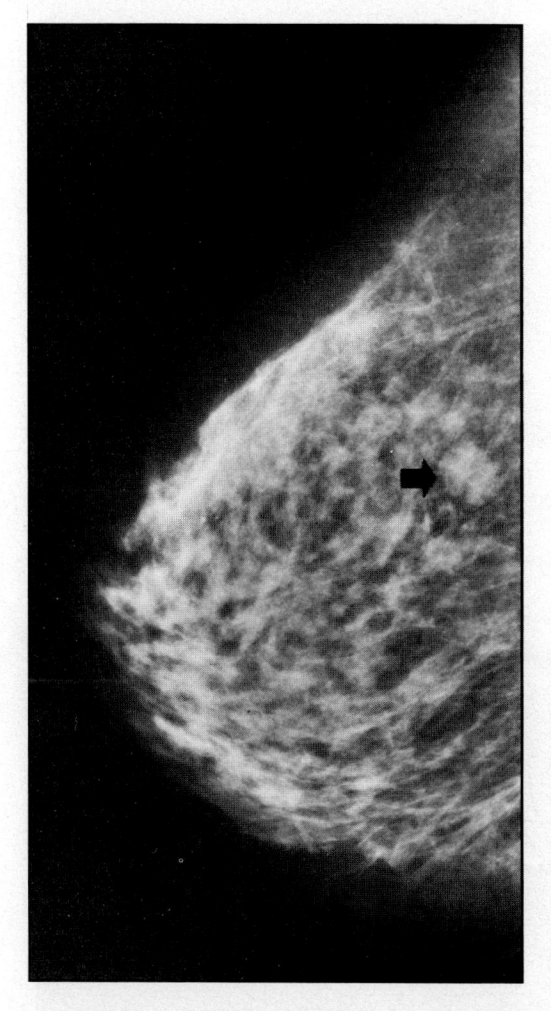

Figure 5-2. Nonpalpable cyst. Routine mammogram depicted mass in this 49-year-old woman.

Figure 5-2A. Mediolateral mammogram reveals prominent ductal pattern and mass in superior hemisphere of right breast (arrow).

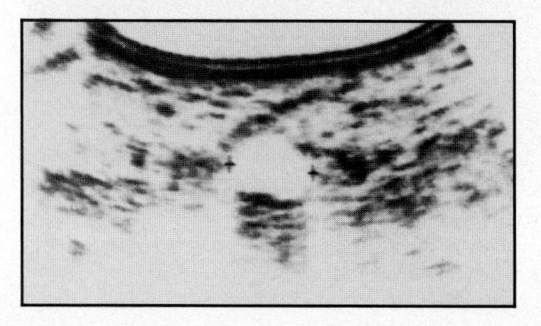

Figure 5-2B. Hand-held real-time examination over area of the mammographic abnormality reveals a 1cm cyst sharply demarcated, anechoic, enhanced distal echoes.

86　breast ultrasound

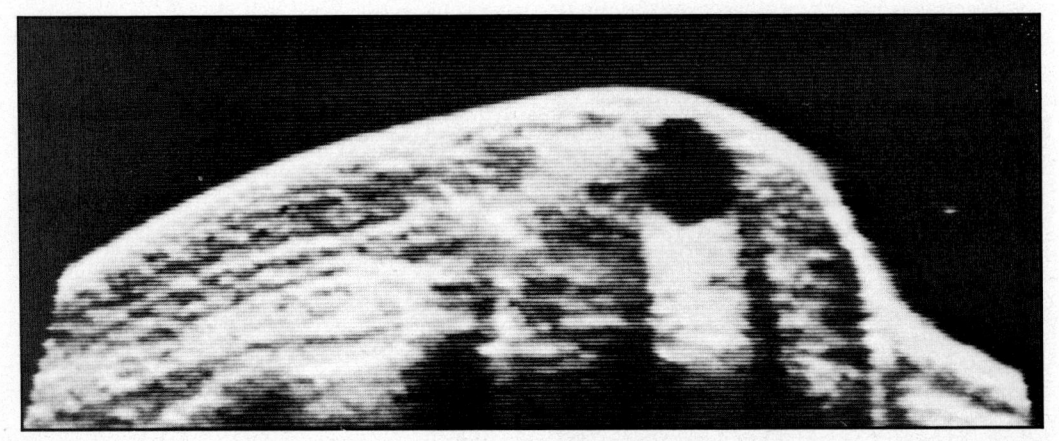

Figure 5-3. A 46-year-old woman with fibrocystic disease and lumpy breasts. Dedicated ultrasound shows cyst, right breast, characterized by anechoic interior, enhanced through-transmission, and lateral capsular refraction. (Technicare)

Figure 5-4. Subareolar cyst, in a 58-year-old woman referred for routine examination.

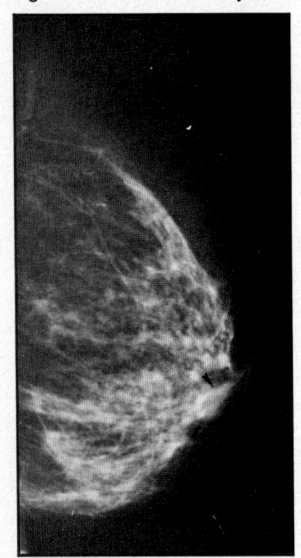

Figure 5-4A. Mediolateral mammogram reveals well-circumscribed subareolar mass (arrowheads).

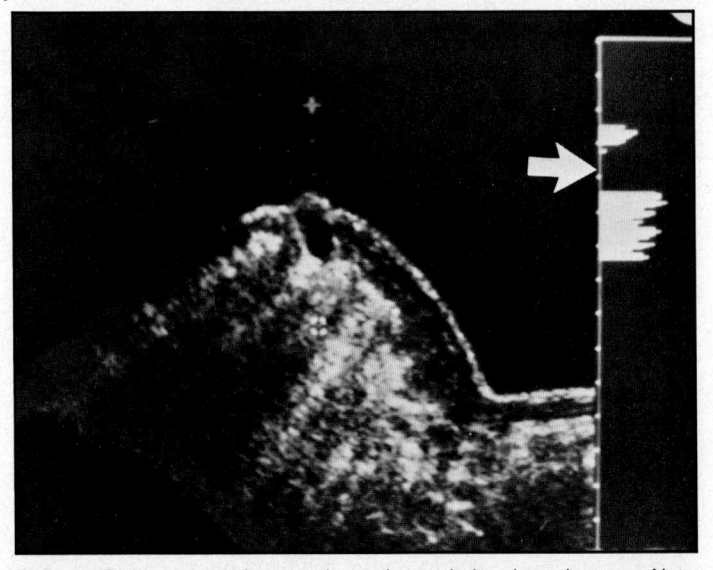

Figure 5-4B. Automated ultrasound reveals anechoic subareolar mass. Note absence of echoes on A-line (arrow), and bright distal echoes. (Ausonics) Diagnosis was cyst; confirmed by needle aspiration.

benign disorders **87**

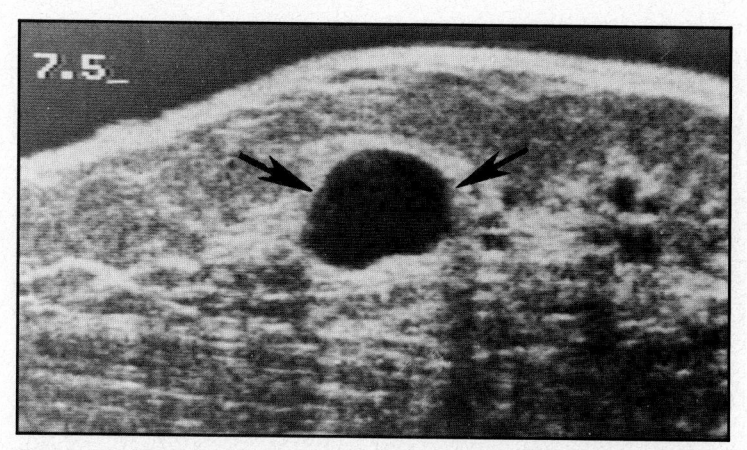

Figure 5-5. One large and several tiny cysts. Characteristic features of large cyst (arrows) are well-defined margins, refractive shadowing off lateral edges of capsule, and enhanced distal echoes. Faint interior echoes are all in anterior-most portion of cyst, a result of high gain setting. (Labsonics) Courtesy of Dr. Elizabeth Kelly-Fry, Indianapolis, Indiana.

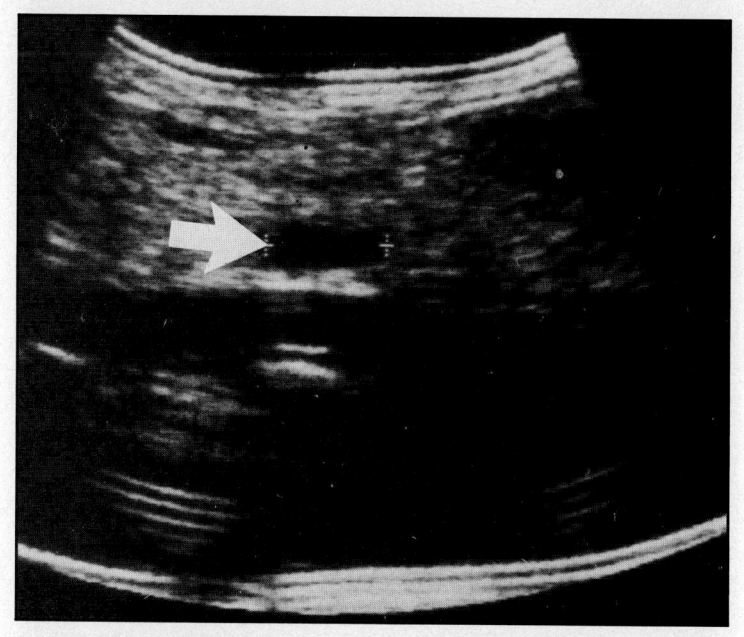

Figure 5-6. Nonpalpable cyst. On real-time examination this sonolucent mass is flattened against chest wall. Chest wall attenuates the through-transmission of echoes. Aspiration under ultrasound guidance confirms cyst.

88 breast ultrasound

Figure 5-7. A 43-year-old woman with multiple palpable masses.

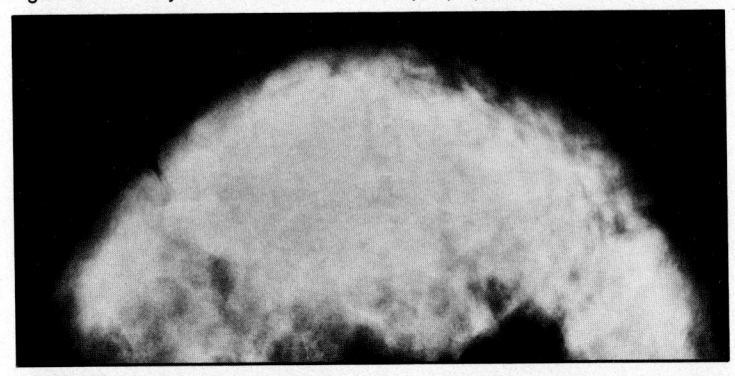

Figure 5-7A. Cephalocaudal mammogram of right breast. Mostly dense tissue with a few well-defined masses.

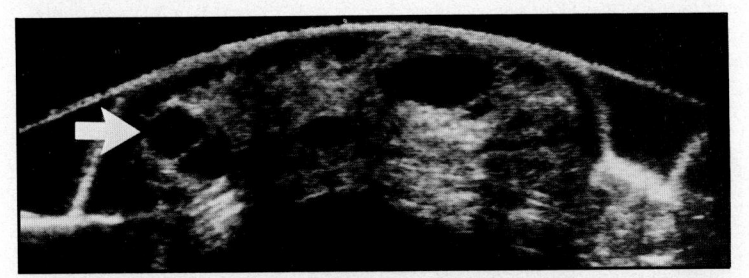

Figure 5-7B. Dedicated ultrasound with compression shows multiple anechoic masses with enhanced acoustic through-transmission. There is a bilobed, septated cyst laterally (arrow). (Ausonics)

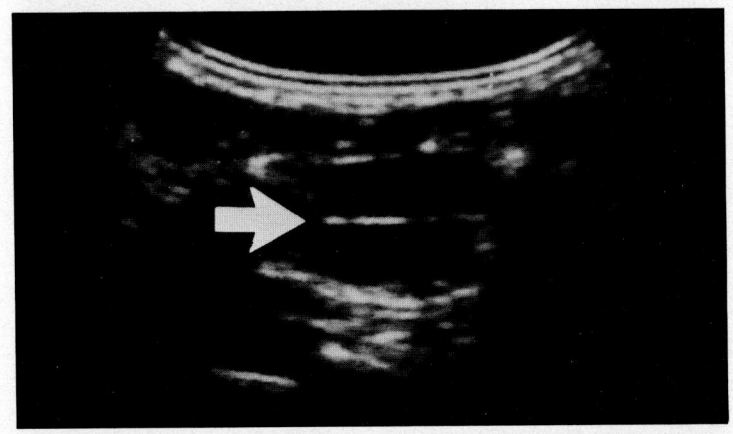

Figure 5-7C. Pressure of manual real-time examination flattens the septated cyst (arrow).

Margins. The anterior and posterior margins of a cyst are usually clearly depicted; however, the curvature of the cyst may make it impossible to visualize its lateral edges, which are specular reflectors. Instead, lateral walls frequently produce posterior refractive shadows beyond the true lateral boundaries of the cysts (Figures 5-3 and 5-5).[4] This refractive shadowing is associated less frequently with benign solid masses such as fibroadenoma.

Shape. Cysts tend to be oval, and may change shape when compression is applied (Figures 5-6 and 5-7C). They may be multiloculated, in which case a smaller cyst may be seen branching from the main cyst. At times, a complete or incomplete septum may be observed within the cyst (Figure 5-7).

Cyst Cavity. The homogeneity of the intracystic fluid is responsible for the anechoic interior of a cyst: its single most important sonographic feature. However, debris in the fluid may occasionally cause internal echoes. The debris is usually found in the most dependent portion of the cyst and may shift when the patient is repositioned. Echoes restricted to the anterior portion of the cyst result from high power settings.

Posterior Enhancement. The enhancement of echoes beyond the cyst is caused by the lower acoustic attenuation coefficient of the cyst relative to that of the surrounding tissues. The resultant "tadpole tail" sign[4] of enhanced posterior echoes is usually present even in association with cysts as small as 3mm. Posterior echo enhancement is better depicted on simple than on compound scans.

Effects on Surrounding Tissues. As the cyst grows, it may alter the sonographic appearance of the surrounding tissues by compressing them. The compressed tissues generally produce stronger than usual echo patterns adjacent to the cyst (Figure 5-1B).

Cyst Aspiration. Ultrasound may be used as a guide for the aspiration of both palpable and nonpalpable cysts.[7]

Multiple Cysts. Multinodular breasts may contain many cysts of varying size. Women with multiple cysts are usually in their thirties or forties, frequently will have undergone multiple biopsies and aspirations, and may have breast pain and tenderness. Ultrasound will depict many cysts of varying size and shape (Figures 5-7). Since ultrasound can show changes in the size of the cysts in response to medical therapy and can be repeated as often as necessary without fear of ionizing radiation, it is an excellent method for follow-up. X-ray mammography is of limited value in these patients because their excessive breast density tends to obscure the cysts, and the x-ray examination cannot distinguish well-circumscribed cystic from solid masses. Nevertheless, annual or biannual x-ray mammography is especially important for women age 40 and older with cystic disease because their breasts are difficult to evaluate by physical examination, and clinically occult cancer may be detectable solely by virtue of the microcalcifications seen in an x-ray mammogram.

FIBROADENOMA

Fibroadenoma is the most frequent tumor of the breast in women under 25 years of age,[8] and is the most common benign solid tumor at any age. This fibroepithelial mass, although usually solitary, is multiple in approximately 15% of cases. Histologically, fibroadenoma is well-encapsulated, and composed of a proliferating fibrous connective tissue stroma surrounding atypical ducts (clefts or acini) lined with epithelium (Figure 5-8). Clinically, it presents as a nontender, rubbery, movable mass. Giant fibroadenoma, usually greater than 10cm in diameter, is a rare variant that occurs almost exclusively in teenagers.[8] During pregnancy fibroadenomas may grow rapidly to a large size. In postmenopausal women, fibroadenomas undergo involution with hyalinization, often resulting in the pathognomonic x-ray mammographic sign of popcorn-like calcifications.

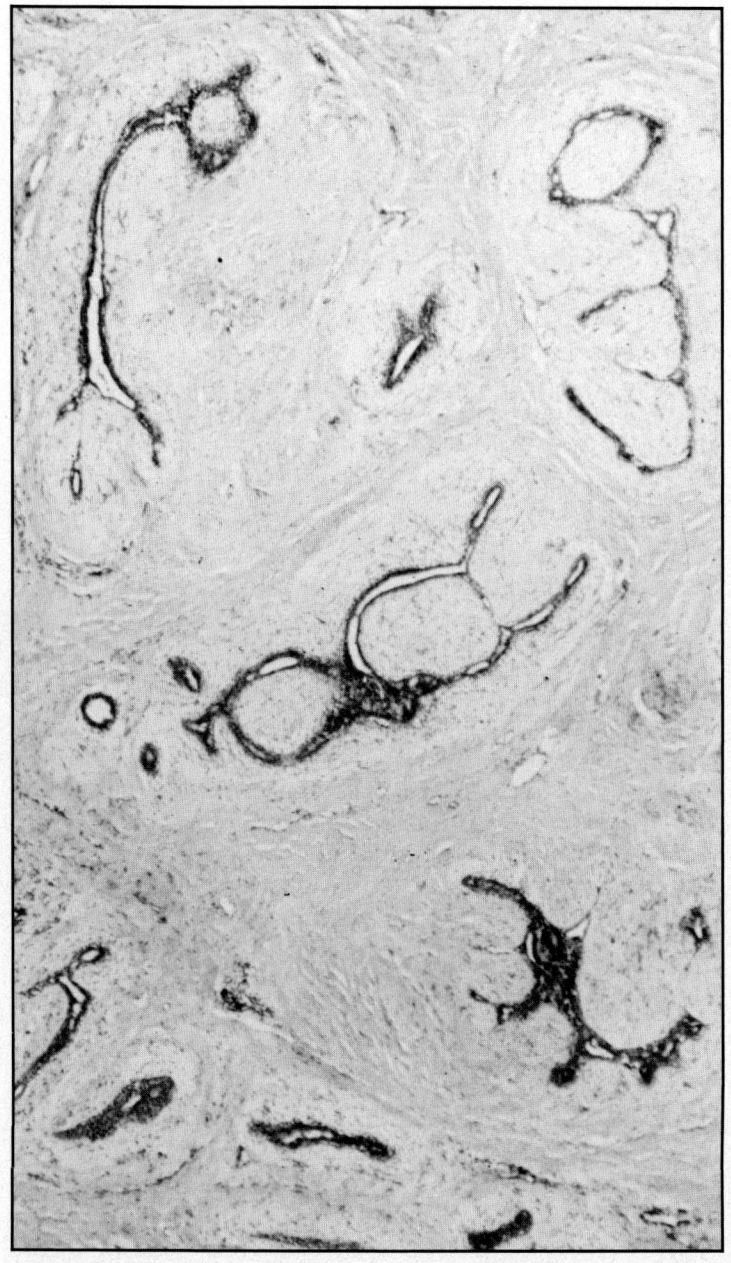

Figure 5-8. Fibroadenoma, histologic section. The benign tumor is composed of fibrous connective tissue and atypical ducts (clefts or acini).

Fibroadenomas are characterized by the following sonographic features: well-circumscribed margins, round to oval shape, uniform internal echoes similar to but usually weaker than those of the surrounding tissues, and posterior echoes that may be moderately diminished, mildly enhanced, or unchanged (Figure 5-9 through 5-13).[2,5]

Margins. The margins are smooth, well demarcated, and sometimes lobulated. Approximately 20% of fibroadenomas show distal refractive shadowing from the edges of the capsule.[9] This refractive edge or lateral shadow sign, more consistently seen with cysts, results from refraction at the lateral aspects of the capsule of the fibroadenoma (Figure 5-9).[4]

Internal Echoes. Characteristic uniform, weak internal echoes, reported to occur in over 80% of fibroadenomas,[10] are attributed to the regular spacing of the epithelial lined clefts within the tumor.

Posterior Attenuation/Enhancement. Fibroadenomas may produce attenuation, enhancement, or no change in posterior echoes. Should attenuation of posterior echoes occur, it is usually only moderate in extent. Enhancement of posterior echoes has been reported in association with about 20% of fibroadenomas (Figure 5-10). With involution and hyalinization there is likely to be even greater distal attenuation of sound (Figure 5-12B).

CYSTOSARCOMA PHYLLOIDES

Cystosarcoma phylloides is a fibroepithelial tumor bearing similarity to and perhaps derivation from fibroadenoma. Cystosarcomas are in general benign, but rarely have been reported to metastasize. Histologically, fibroadenoma has a hypocellular fibrous connective tissue stroma, while cystosarcoma manifests an excessively cellular, often sarcoma-like stroma. The usual sonographic features of cystosarcoma include well-defined borders, generally low-

benign disorders   **93**

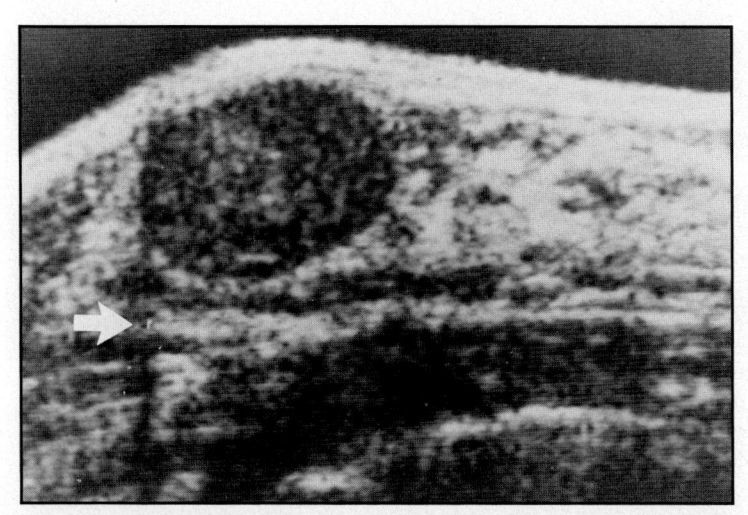

Figure 5-9. Fibroadenoma, in an 18-year-old with palpable mass. Note sharp boundaries, homogeneous interior echo pattern and thin refractive shadows (arrow) from lateral aspects of capsule. (Labsonics) Courtesy of Dr. Elizabeth Kelly-Fry, Indianapolis, Indiana.

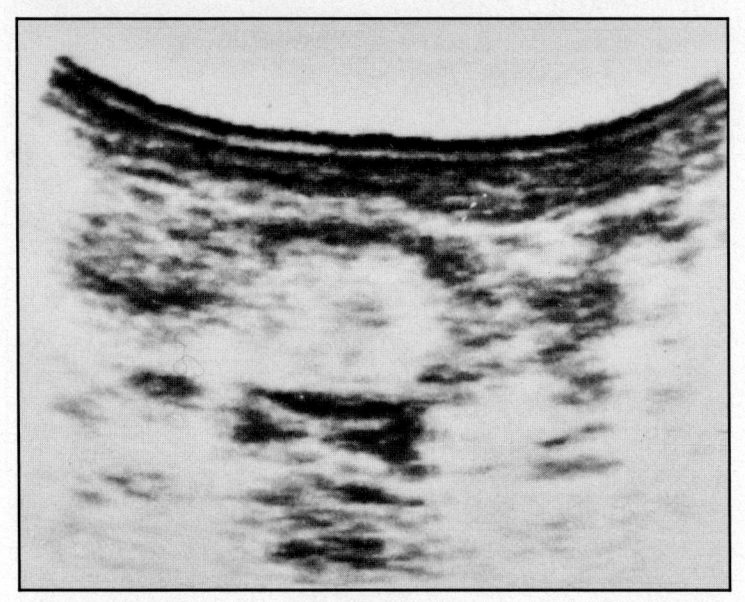

Figure 5-10. Fibroadenoma. A 30-year-old woman with lump in left breast for 4 months. Hand-held real-time examination reveals well-defined mass with even echoes of low intensity in comparison to surrounding parenchyma, and enhanced distal echoes.

94 breast ultrasound

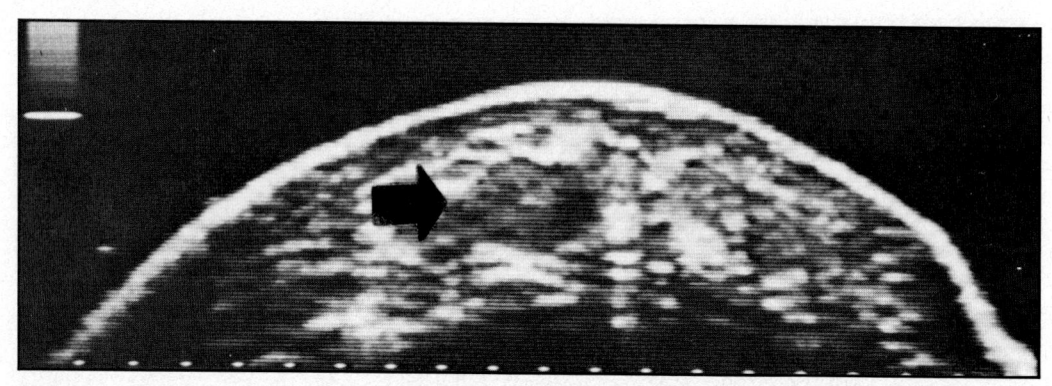

Figure 5-11. A 24-year-old with thickening in left breast at 12:00. Dedicated ultrasound reveals mass with smooth contour and homogeneous low-level internal echoes (arrow). (Technicare) Biopsy revealed fibroadenoma. Courtesy of Louise S. O'Shaughnessy, MD, San Diego, California.

Figure 5-12. A 37-year-old woman with palpable mass, right breast.

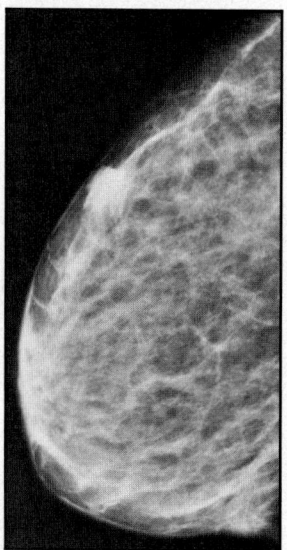

Figure 5-12A. Mediolateral mammogram shows well-defined density, upper hemisphere.

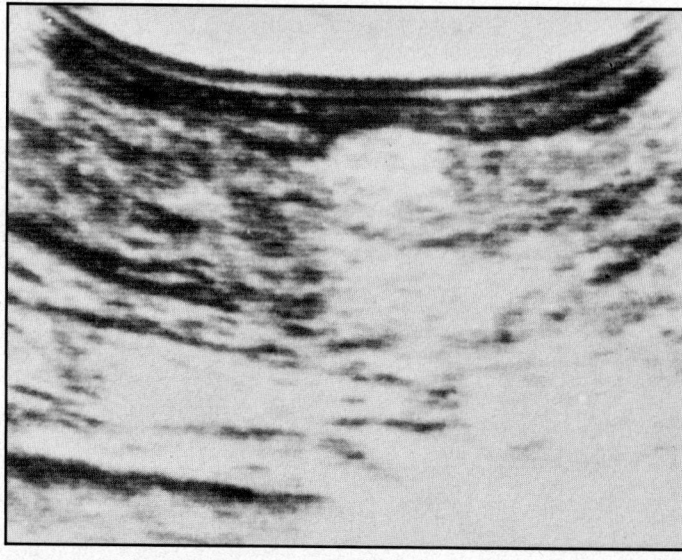

Figure 5-12B. Hand-held examination shows well-defined mass abuting the skin but not affecting subcutaneous echoes. There is distal echo attenuation. Biopsy revealed fibroadenoma.

level interior echoes, and moderately enhanced posterior echoes (Figure 5-14). The enhanced through-transmission of sound associated with cystosarcoma may be due to the presence of fluid-filled cystic spaces within the tumor.[11]

INTRADUCTAL PAPILLOMA

A papilloma is a benign epithelial tumor composed of a central stalk of connective tissue covered by epithelial cells.[12] The average age of patients with symptomatic papilloma is approximately 40 years. Papillomas arise within ducts, usually a major duct near the nipple or one of its large branches, and may be single or multiple. The most frequent symptom is a bloody or serous discharge from the nipple. In fact, papilloma is the most frequent cause, benign or malignant, of a bloody discharge. Ultrasound may occasionally depict the intraluminal filling defect (Figure 5-15).[13]

LIPOMA

Lipomas tend to be found most often in the atrophic breasts of postmenopausal women. They are solitary, slow growing, and asymptomatic. On physical examination they are soft and movable. Their palpable margins may be difficult to discern from the equally soft texture of surrounding fatty breast tissue. Lipomas are recognized on mammograms as a mass of radiolucent fat with a thin, smooth, well-defined capsule of water-density (Figure 5-16A).

The sonographic appearance of a lipoma depends on the nature of the surrounding breast tissue. If the wall of the lipoma is visible, it appears smooth. Within a dense breast, the lipoma appears circumscribed, with internal echoes that are weak relative to the surrounding parenchyma. Distal echoes may be enhanced or normal. In a fatty breast, a small lipoma is difficult to appreciate on the ultrasound image because its echoes are similar to those of the surrounding fat. Since the acoustic absorption of the fat

96 breast ultrasound

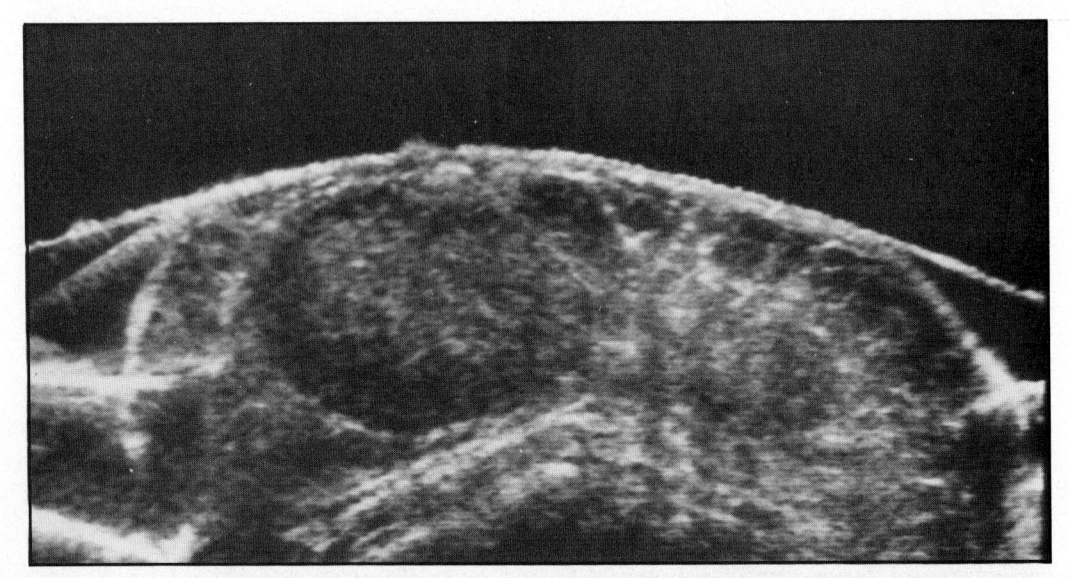

Figure 5-13. Large fibroadenoma of pregnancy. This 25-year-old woman felt firm mass in her left breast during sixth month of pregnancy. Whole-breast automated ultrasound with compression shows a well-circumscribed mass with homogeneous medium-level echoes.

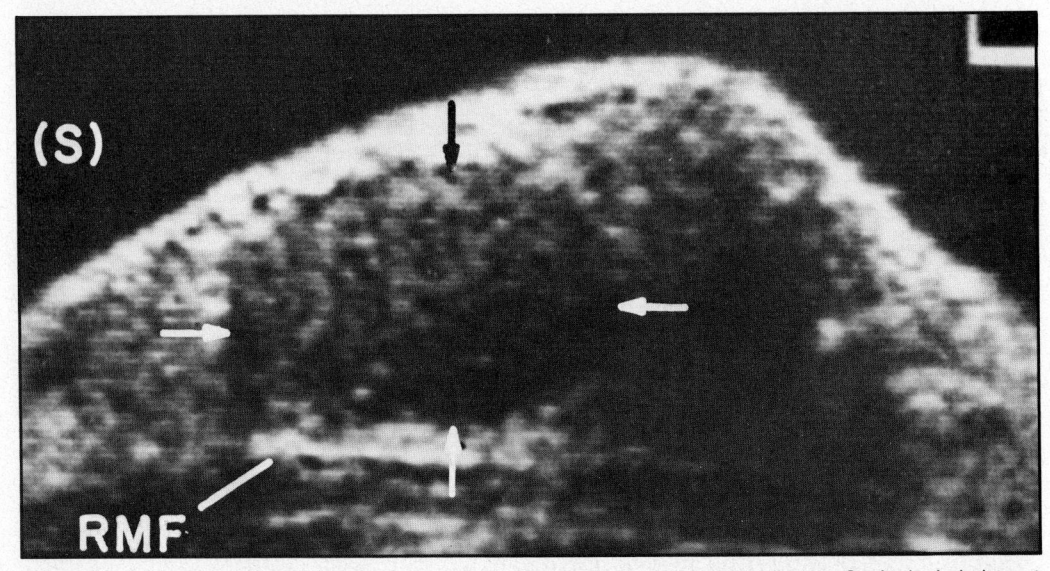

Figure 5-14. A 17-year-old woman had a palpable 6cm mass in the left superior breast. Sagittal whole-breast scan shows a superior (S) solid mass (arrows) with lobulated margins, weak internal echoes, and moderate through-transmission of sound. RMF = retromammary fat. (Technicare) Courtesy of Catherine Cole-Beuglet, MD Irvine, California

benign disorders 97

Figure 5-15. Intraductal papilloma, in a 39-year-old woman with 16-year history of nipple discharge. *From Rubin: AJR 144:623-627, 1985.*

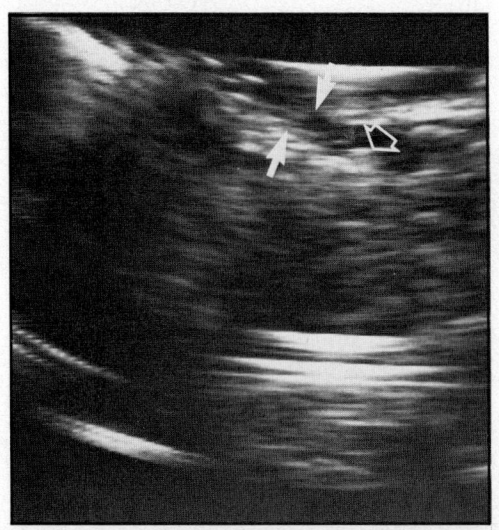

Figure 5-15A. Sonogram obtained with water-path step-off device, causing broad echoes in near field. Dilated ducts (arrows) extend to nipple. On real-time examination there was a persistent intraluminal filling defect (open arrow).

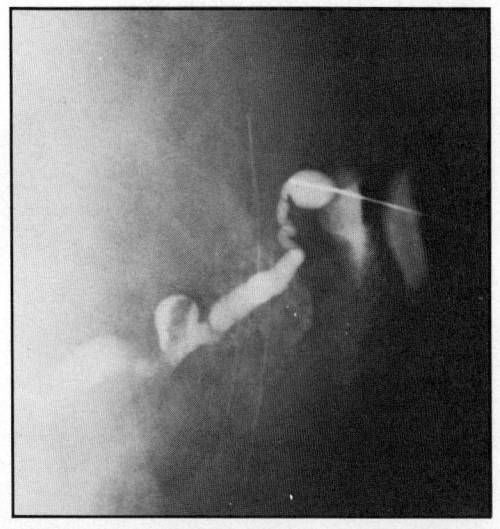

Figure 5-15B. Lateral ductogram. Tortuous dilated duct with at least two round intraluminal papillomas.

Figure 5-16. Lipoma. A 60-year-old woman noticed soft mass under the nipple of left breast.

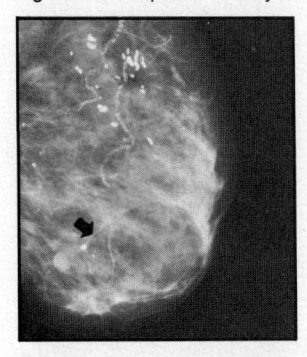

Figure 5-16A. Oblique view film-screen mammogram showed benign calcifications in upper part of breast, radiolucent encapsulated lipoma at the palpable abnormality (arrow), and small cyst posterior to lipoma.

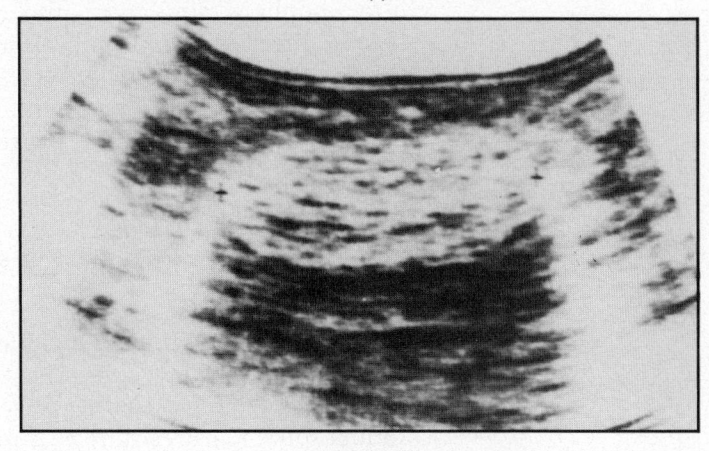

Figure 5-16B. Hand-held real-time ultrasound of lipoma shows well-circumscribed mass with lateral edge refraction, low-level internal echoes, and enhanced through-transmission.

98 breast ultrasound

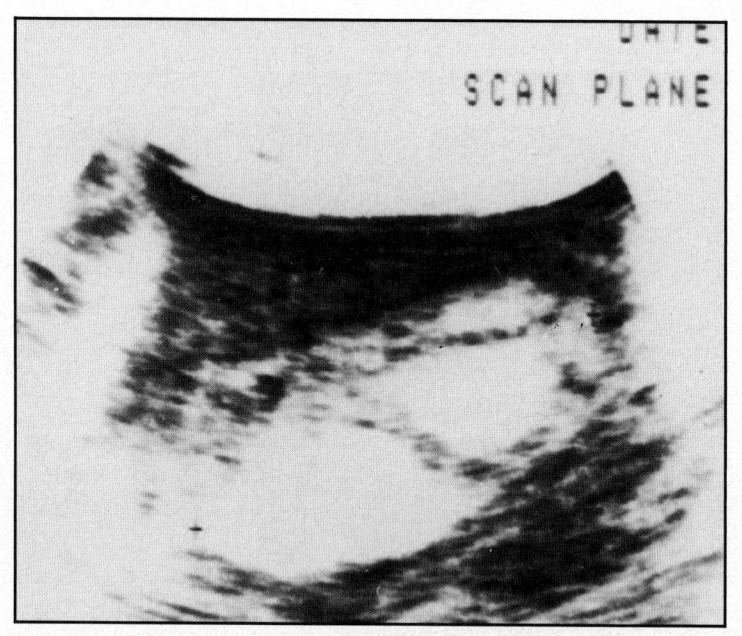

Figure 5-17. A 38-year-old woman complained of breast pain, subareolar mass, and fever. Hand-held real-time examination of subareolar tissues depicts multilobulated mass with a few low-level interior echoes.

of a lipoma is similar to that of the surrounding fatty tissue, there is usually no appreciable enhancement or attenuation of posterior echoes. However, if the lipoma is large, distinctive low-level echoes, refractive shadowing from the capsule, and/or distal echo attenuation may be identified (Figure 5-16B).

ABSCESS

A typical clinical history includes fever, pain, tenderness, and an enlarging mass. Abscesses are found frequently in the subareolar region. Since abscesses contain fluid, their sonographic features may be similar to those of cysts. An abscess is typically characterized by a well-defined anechoic region with thick irregular walls, and frequently multiple septations (Figure 5-17).

GALACTOCELE

A galactocele arises in the lactating breast, and represents a localized accumulation of milk resulting from an obstructed duct. It is usually detected long after nursing has been terminated. Galactoceles may have sonographic features similar to those of cysts, with oval shape and well delimited margins. However, its inspissated milk content gives rise to multiple low-level echoes. Posterior enhancement, when present, is moderate (Figure 5-18).

SEBACEOUS CYST

A sebaceous cyst in the skin of the breast is identified by its superficial location, fluid content, and circumscribed character (Figure 5-19).

HEMATOMA

An acute hematoma is usually characterized sonographically as a poorly defined focus of architectural disruption that contains weak internal echoes (Figure 5-20).[14] There is frequently a history of trauma or surgery immediately preceding the onset of the mass. The hematoma may liquify within two or three hours of its onset, leading to an alternate sonographic appearance of a fluid-filled area that is slow to resolve (Figure 5-21).

OTHER BIOPSY CHANGES

Following biopsy of the breast, changes occur in the skin and in the texture of the parenchyma. The skin may become thickened and retracted at the site of the incision. Parenchymal scars may attenuate the sonic beam. Therefore, it is important to be aware of the sites of previous biopsies when interpreting the sonographic examination.

100   breast ultrasound

Figure 5-18. A 32-year-old woman, 3 months postpartum, has a persistent lump in lower-inner quadrant of left breast.

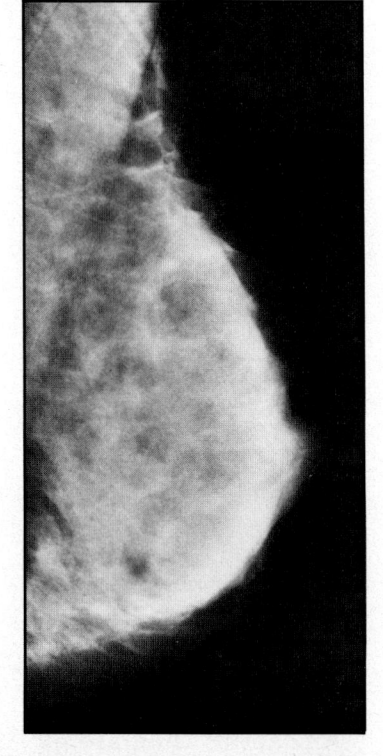

Figure 5-18A. Mediolateral mammogram shows no abnormalities.

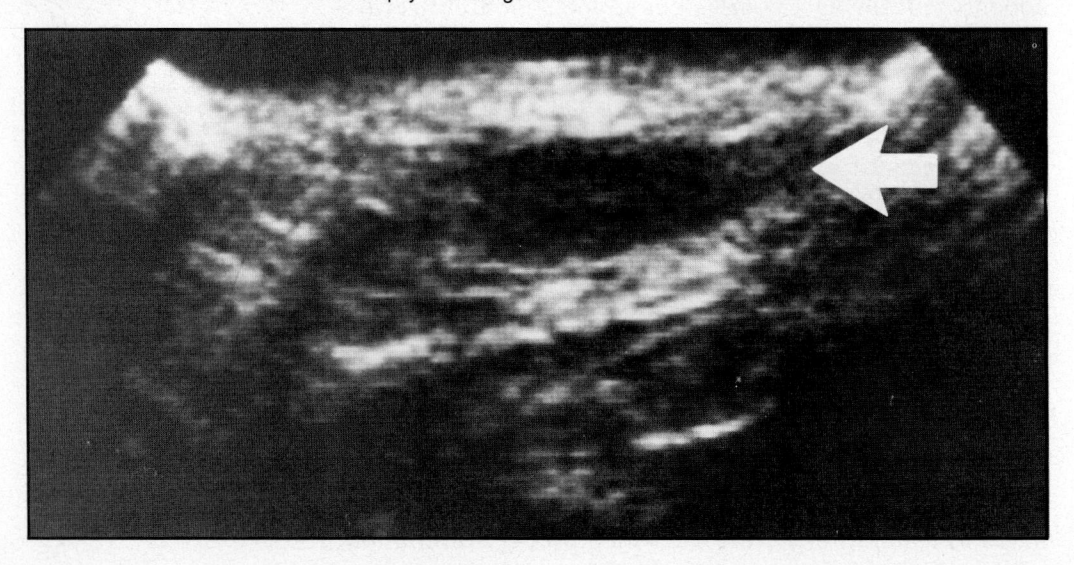

Figure 5-18B. Hand-held real-time examination shows pliable well-defined mass with fine internal echoes. Biopsy revealed galactocele.

benign disorders 101

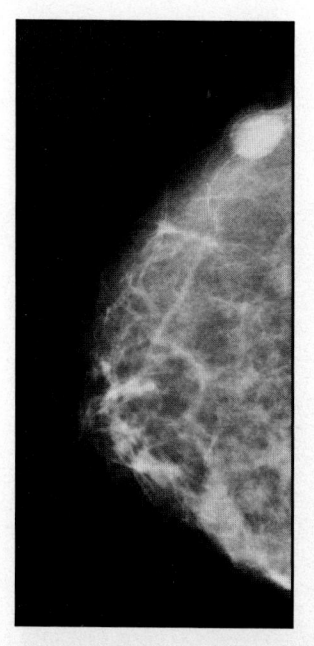

Figure 5-19. Sebaceous cyst. A 46-year-old woman with small lump in right breast.

Figure 5-19A. Mediolateral mammogram shows 2cm well-circumscribed mass in upper hemisphere.

Figure 5-19B. Hand-held real-time ultrasound shows well-circumscribed cyst-like mass with small amount of debris at dependent portion. Biopsy confirmed sebaceous cyst.

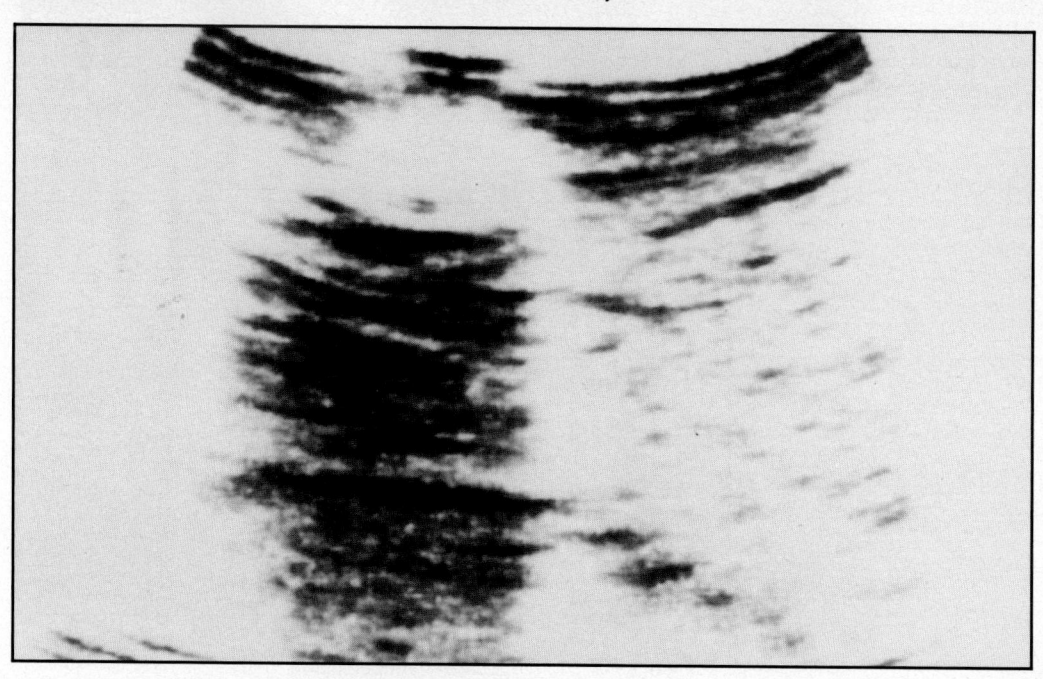

102   breast ultrasound

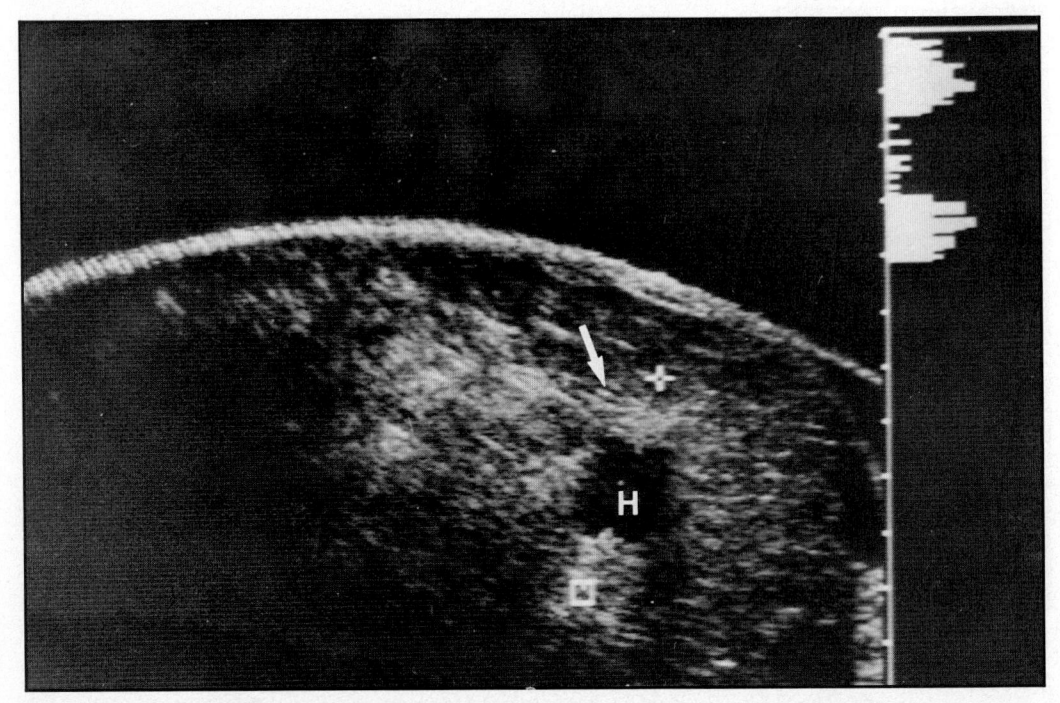

Figure 5-20. Acute hematoma (H) is hypoechoic and causes compression of the surrounding tissue (arrow). From McSweeney: Radiol Cl North Am 23:157, 1985.

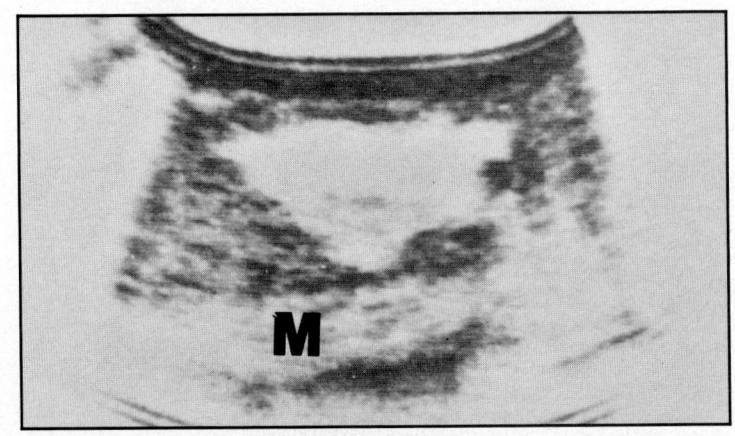

Figure 5-21. Liquifying hematoma, two weeks following biopsy of fibroadenoma. Sediment settling to most dependent portion. M = pectoralis muscle.

benign disorders **103**

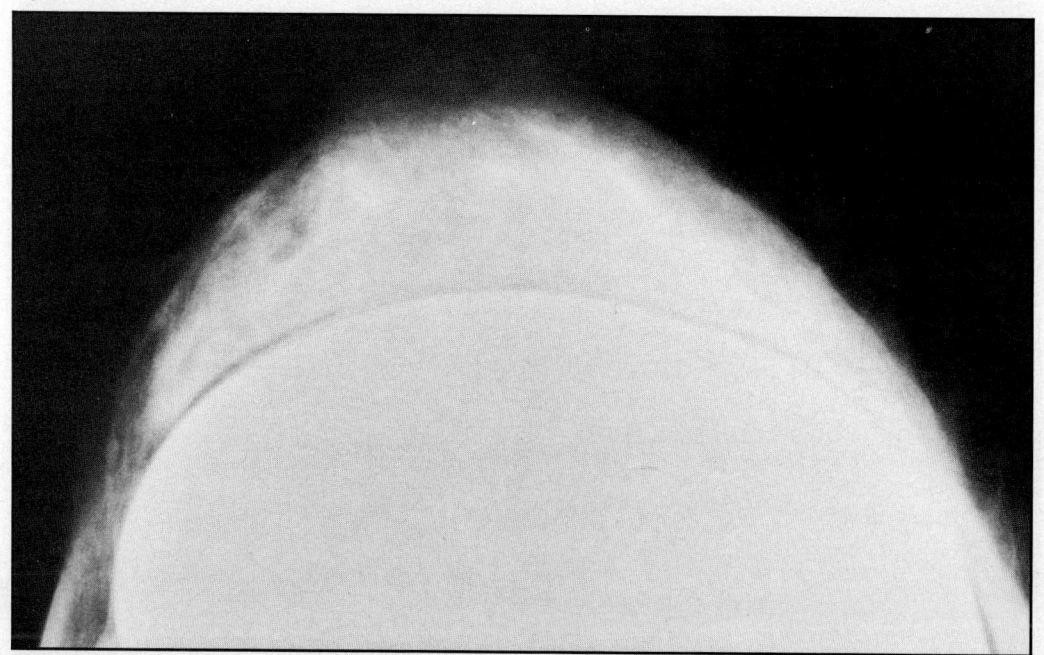

Figure 5-22.

Figure 5-22A. Cephalocaudal mammogram shows dense silicone-gel implant in breast.

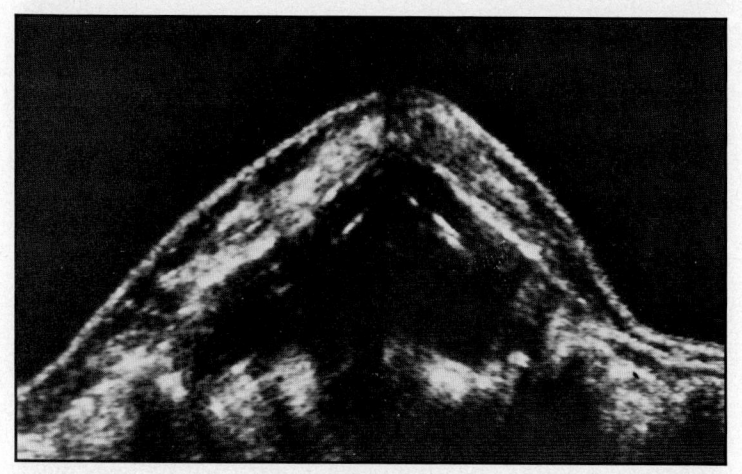

Figure 5-22B. Ultrasound shows implant depicted as well-circumscribed central region of diminished echoes. (Ausonics)

104 breast ultrasound

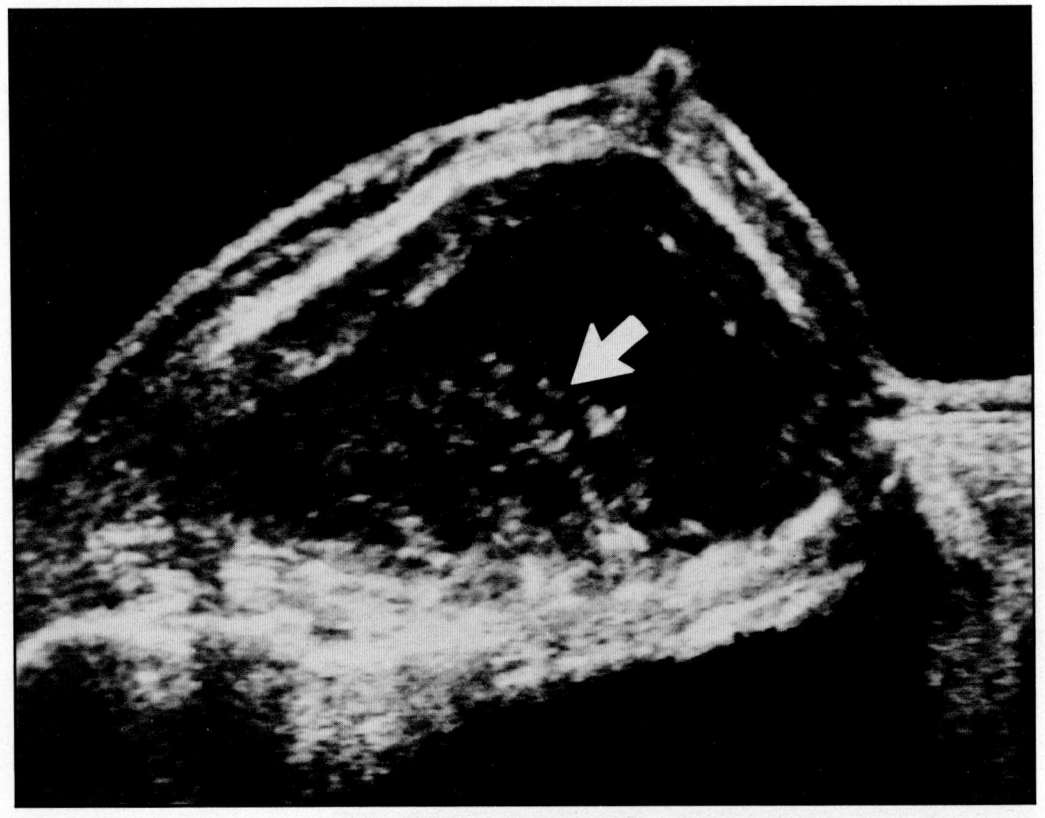

Figure 5-23. Debris (arrow) within this implant changed position when patient was moved. (Ausonics)

BREAST AUGMENTATION MAMMOPLASTY

Saline or silicone gel-filled bag implants are the most common augmentation prostheses. Although they tend to limit the usefulness of both x-ray and ultrasound mammographic examinations, ultrasound sometimes depicts more of the displaced breast tissue. The prosthetic bag usually appears as a relatively echo-free area in the center of the breast (Figure 5-22). It is not unusual, however, to see debris within the prosthesis (Figure 5-23). Ultrasound has been reported to be useful in evaluating complications

benign disorders **105**

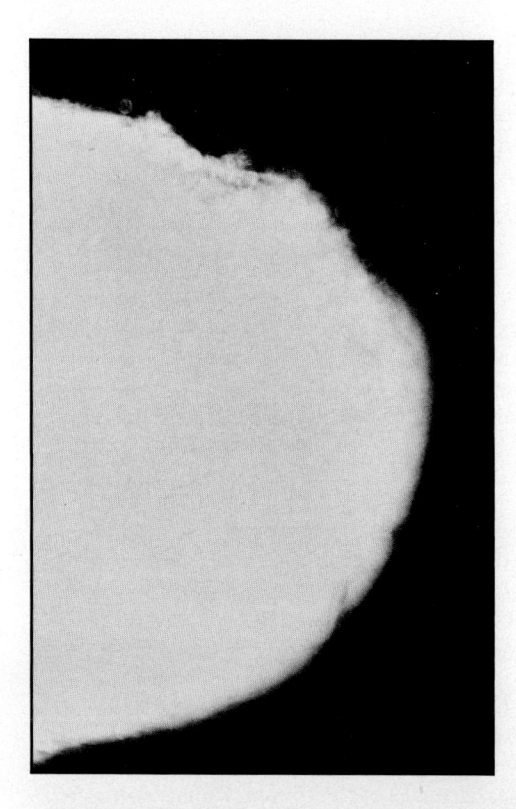

Figure 5-24. A 48-year-old woman who had cosmetic silicone injections years ago now feels many lumps.

Figure 5-24A. Mediolateral mammogram. Breast is totally opacified.

Figure 5-24B. Silicone attenuates most of the sound. (Ausonics)

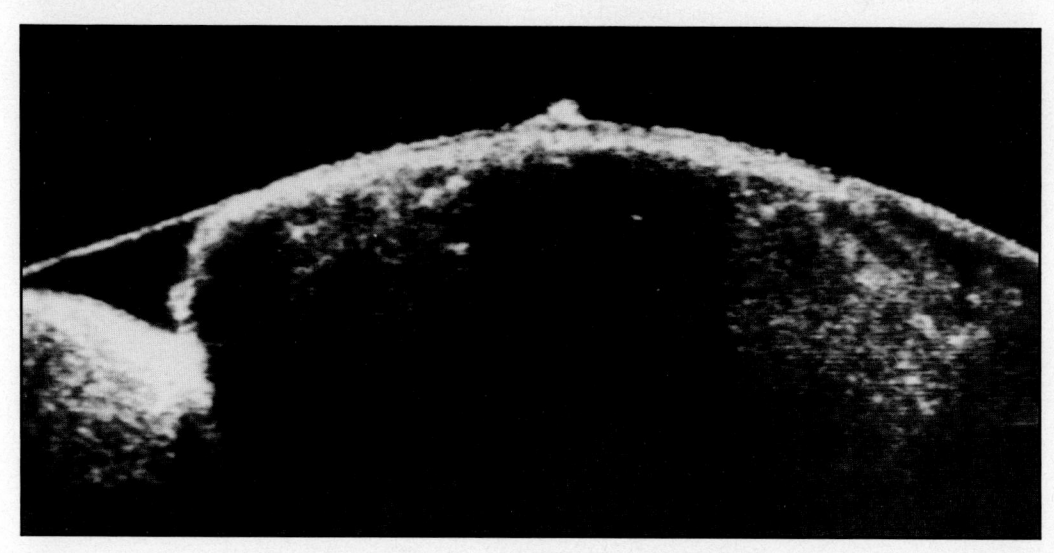

of mammoplasty, such as abscess formation, displacement of implants, and fibrous capsule formation.[15] Injected silicone causes combinations of shadowing and increased through-transmission, and, as in x-ray mammography, it severely limits the diagnostic value of the ultrasound examination (Figure 5-24).

References

1. Haagensen CD: Diseases of the Breast. Philadelphia: W.B. Saunders, 1971, p 155.
2. Jellins J, Kossoff G, Reeve TS: Detection and classification of liquid-filled masses in the breast by gray scale echography. Radiology 125:205-212, 1977.
3. Sickles EA, Filly RA, Callen PW: Benign breast lesions: ultrasound detection and diagnosis. Radiology 151:467-470, 1984.
4. Kobayashi T, Takatani O, Hattori N, et al: Differential diagnosis of breast tumors. Cancer 33:940-951, 1974.
5. Cole-Beuglet C, Beique RA: Continuous ultrasound B-scanning of palpable breast masses. Radiology 117:123-128, 1975.
6. Baum G: Ultrasound mammography. Radiology 122:199-205, 1977.
7. Kopans DB: Breast ultrasound. *In* Feig SA (ed): Syllabus for the Categorical Course on Mammography. Chicago: American College of Radiology, 1984, p 173.
8. Haagensen CD: Diseases of the Breast. Philadelphia: W.B. Saunders, 1971, p 212.
9. Egan RL, Egan KL: Automated water-path full-breast sonography: correlation with histology of 176 solid lesions. AJR 143:499-507, 1984.
10. Cole-Beuglet C, Soriano RZ, Kurtz AB, Goldberg BB: Fibroadenoma of the breast: sonomammography correlated with pathology in 122 patients. AJR 140:369-375, 1983.
11. Cole-Beuglet C, Soriano R, Kurtz AB, Meyer JE, Kopans DB, Goldberg BB: Ultrasound, x-ray mammogrphy, and histopathology of cystosarcoma phylloides. Radiology 146:481-486, 1983.
12. Cutler M: Tumors of the Breast. Philadelphia: J.B. Lippincott, 1962, p. 83.
13. Rubin E, Miller VE, Berland LL, et al: Real-time breast sonography. AJR 144:623-627, 1985.
14. McSweeney MB, Murphy CH: Whole-breast sonography. Radiol Clin North Am 23:157-167, 1985.
15. Cole-Beuglet C, Schwartz G, Kurtz AB, Patchefsky AS, Goldberg BB: Ultrasound mammography for the augmented breast. Radiology 146:737-742, 1983.

CHAPTER 6

Malignant Lesions

INTRODUCTION

This chapter presents the sonographic features of breast malignancies. While x-ray mammography is a superior technique for breast cancer screening,[1] sonomammography is a useful adjunct in the evaluation of breast lumps, especially in the dense breast. Occasionally, whole-breast ultrasound is the only method that reveals a cancer in a breast that is dense in x-ray mammograms. In a dense breast the cancer is characterized by an area of low-level echoes, possibly with posterior shadowing, within a background of uniform, high-level parenchymal echoes.[2] However, in a sonogram of a fatty breast, a cancer may be difficult to identify because the surrounding fat is also low in echogenicity.

The ultrasound appearances of the various types of breast carcinoma are not consistent enough to accurately predict their histology. Rather, they manifest a broad range of sonographic features. Infiltrating ductal carcinoma tends to have the most characteristically malignant features, while medullary carcinoma tends to have features similar to those of benign solid masses. Carcinoma masses may be conveniently classified sonographically according to the extent of circumscription of their margins.

Following a presentation of the general ultrasound features of poorly circumscribed and well circumscribed carcinomas, we will address the features of specific histologic types of carcinoma.

ULTRASOUND FEATURES OF BREAST CARCINOMAS

Poorly Circumscribed Carcinomas

Infiltrating ductal carcinoma, the most common breast malignancy, usually forms a mass that is poorly circumscribed. In x-ray mammograms the majority of these tumors are dense, have irregular or spiculated margins, and may be associated with microcalcifications and adjacent parenchymal and skin changes. Histologically, they contain a preponderance of fibrous connective tissue in comparison

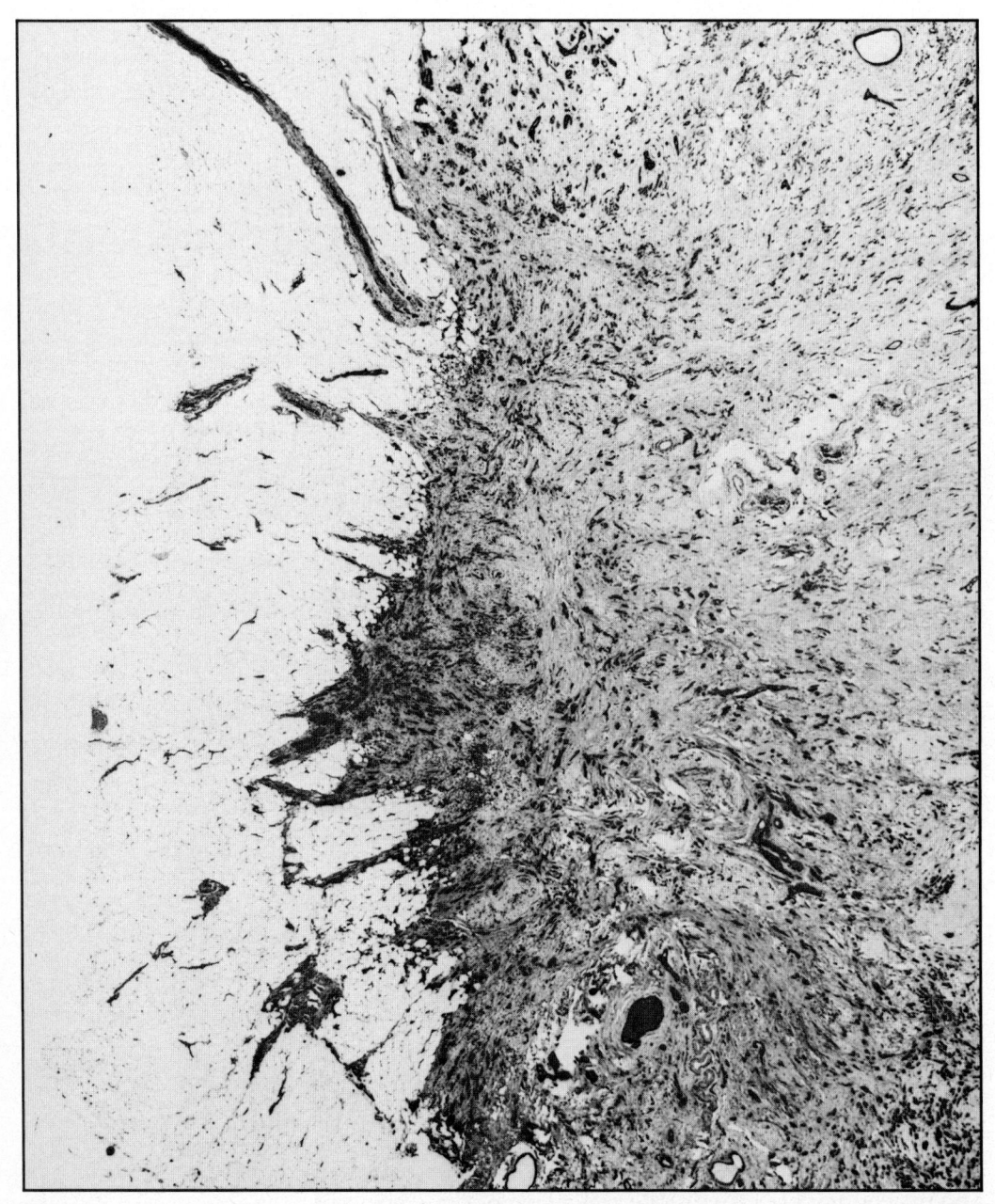

Figure 6-1. Margin of infiltrating ductal carcinoma. Histologic section. Cellularity is much less prominent than large amount of fibrous stroma. Note irregular, highly infiltrative tumor margin (hematoxylin and eosin stain, ×10).

to the far lesser extent of epithelial tumor cells (Figure 6-1).[3] The primary sonographic signs of poorly circumscribed infiltrating carcinomas are: irregular margins; moderately sharp anterior boundary but poor-to-absent posterior boundary; weak, inhomogeneous internal echoes; and lack of posterior echoes (Figures 6-2 through 6-6).[3-7] Secondary signs include alteration of the surrounding breast architecture, thickening and/or straightening of Cooper's ligaments, skin thickening and retraction or flattening, and alteration of the subcutaneous fat (Figures 6-5B and 6-6B).[8] Microcalcifications, often the key feature of this tumor in x-ray mammograms and especially of lesions 1 cm or less in diameter, are not usually imaged in sonograms. Thus x-ray mammography is far more accurate in early diagnosis than sonography.

Margins. Infiltrating ductal carcinoma has a jagged, uneven, boundary.[4] The boundary echoes are usually intermediate in brightness anteriorly and weak to absent posteriorly. The ability to define the margin depends both on the nature of the lesion and the angle of incidence of the ultrasound beam. The medial and lateral borders of the tumor are usually better visualized than its anterior and posterior borders. Because the boundary echoes of highly infiltrating carcinoma may be difficult to identify, the extent of the lesion must often be assumed from the appearance of the contrasting surrounding echoes.

Internal Echoes. The internal echoes of infiltrating ductal carcinoma may vary in intensity from one tumor to the next, but generally are of a low level, similar to those of fatty tissue, and lower than those of breast parenchymal tissue. The echoes are often nonuniform in size and intensity within the tumor.

Posterior Echoes. Shadowing or attenuation of posterior echoes is an important sign of malignancy that occurs in approximately two-thirds of infiltrating carcinomas.[5] This sign has also been termed posterior shadowing, posterior attenuation, distal shadowing, distal attenuation,

112 *breast ultrasound*

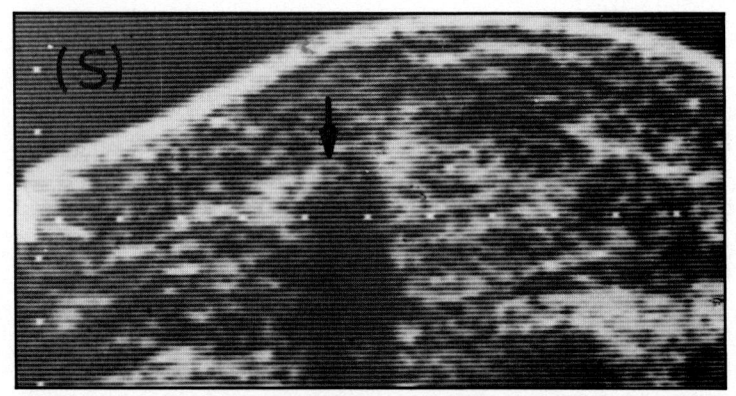

Figure 6-2. Dedicated ultrasound, sagittal section, shows superior (S) hypoechoic mass (arrow) with poorly defined margins and distal shadowing. (Technicare) Biopsy revealed infiltrating ductal carcinoma. Courtesy of Catherine Cole-Beuglet, MD, Irvine, California.

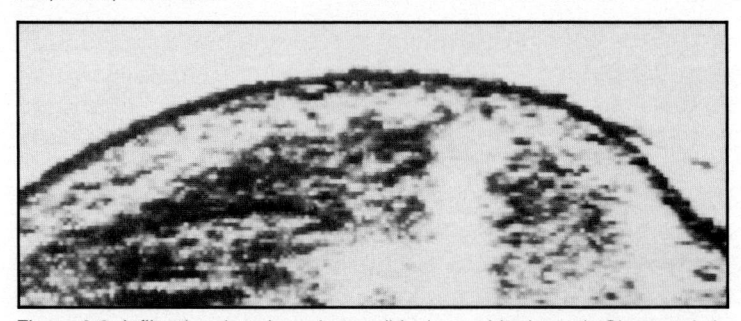

Figure 6-3. Infiltrative ductal carcinoma (black on white image). Characteristic features are poorly-defined margins, inhomogeneous low-level echoes compared to surrounding parenchyma, and striking lack of sound posterior to mass. (Technicare) Courtesy of Edward A. Sickles, MD, San Francisco, California.

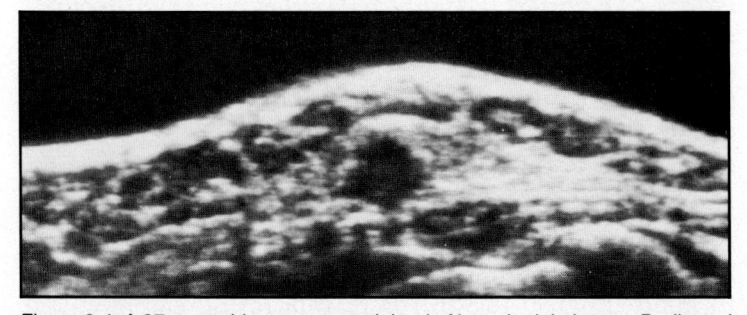

Figure 6-4. A 37-year-old woman complained of lump in right breast. Dedicated ultrasound shows mass with irregular borders and uneven internal echoes. Biopsy revealed infiltrating ductal carcinoma. (Labsonics) Courtesy of Wende W. Logan, MD, Buffalo, New York.

retrotumorous shadowing, and acoustic middle shadowing. The phenomenon of a lack of posterior echoes is believed to be due to the high absorption of ultrasonic energy by the tumor. Kobayashi[9] and Cole-Beuglet[3] independently reported that the degree of distal echo attenuation was directly proportional to the fibrous connective tissue content of the tumor, generally being greatest in infiltrating ductal carcinoma. Egan,[10] however, found that the lack of distal echoes, as well as irregularity of tumor margin and internal echo content, was more consistently related to the signs of invasiveness found in x-ray mammograms than to the degree of desmoplasia or fibrosis found histologically.

Secondary Signs. Alteration and disruption of the sonographic image of the surrounding parenchyma is frequently observed in association with infiltrating carcinoma. This includes a halo of low level echo intensity that often surrounds the tumor. The parenchymal changes are most obvious in dense breasts, where the echo intensity of the normal parenchyma is relatively high.

Changes in skin contour and thickness are best visualized in examinations performed with water-path automated scanners. Skin thickening may cause the appearance of a double line of echoes at the water-skin interface.[11]

Bilateral asymmetry of the ultrasonic penetration of the breasts is as important a clue to possible malignancy as is the asymmetry in parenchymal density found in x-ray mammography.[12] Lack of penetration of an area in one breast should be viewed with suspicion, and a further attempt should be made to depict the region by increasing sonic power and/or by using breast compression.

Focal abnormalities may be present in the subcutaneous fat overlying a carcinoma. The fat may become more echogenic and the normally well demarcated fat-parenchymal interface may be lost (Figure 6-6B).

Well-Circumscribed Carcinomas

The approximately 10% of breast carcinoma masses that have a well-circumscribed margin on ultrasound images[8] are often difficult or impossible to differentiate

Figure 6-5. A 43-year-old woman complained of "tugging" sensation above left nipple.

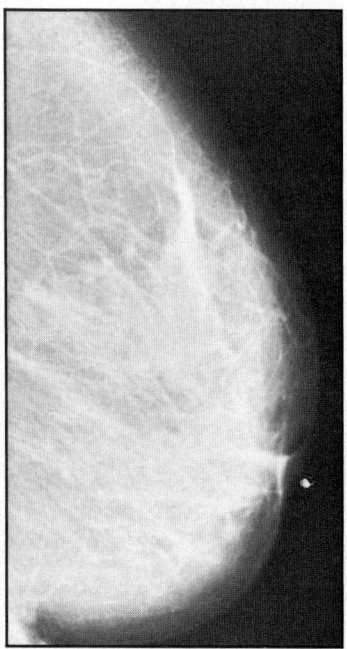

Figure 6-5A. Mediolateral mammogram shows nipple retraction.

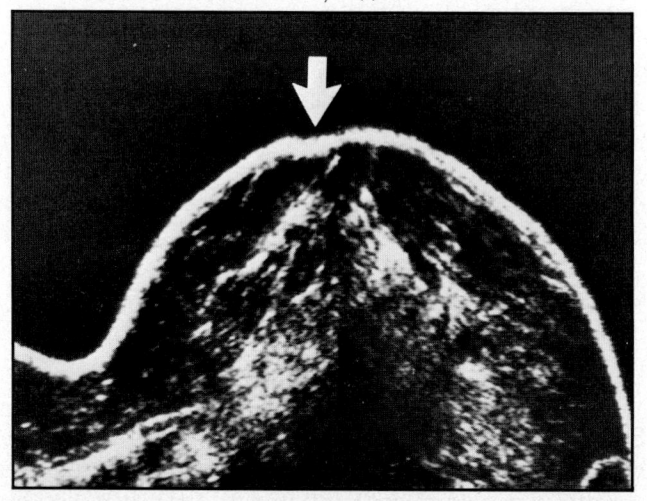

Figure 6-5B. Whole-breast ultrasound. Transverse section of noncompressed left breast (split-screen image: right half from one transducer; left half from opposing transducer) shows skin retraction (arrow). (Ausonics)

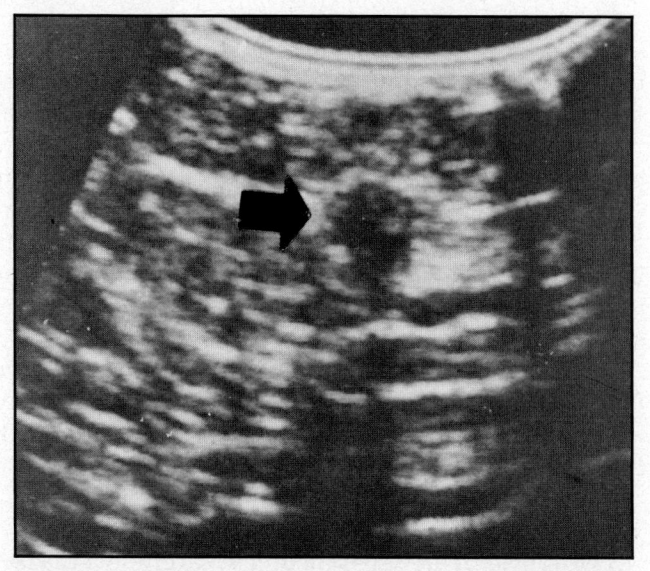

Figure 6-5C. Hand-held real-time ultrasound shows hypoechoic mass with fairly sharp anterior margin but poor posterior margin. Mass attenuates distal echoes. Biopsy revealed infiltrating ductal carcinoma.

malignant lesions 115

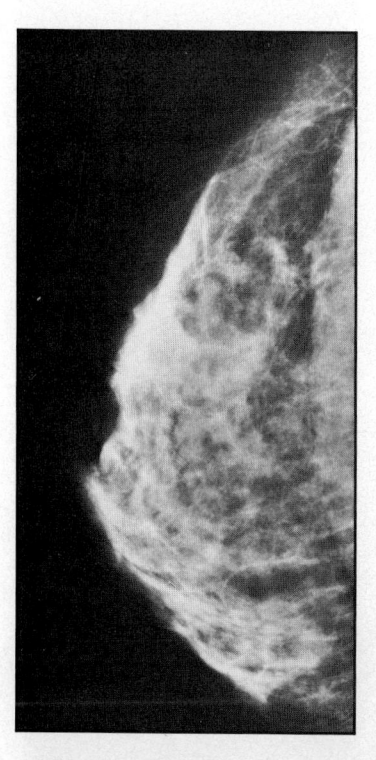

Figure 6-6. A 39-year-old woman with family history of breast carcinoma felt mass in right breast above nipple.

Figure 6-6A. Mediolateral mammogram was negative.

Figure 6-6B. Sagittal section (split-screen) at nipple showed hypoechoic mass above nipple. Adjacent subcutaneous fat (arrow) and surrounding parenchymal echo patterns are disrupted. (Ausonics)

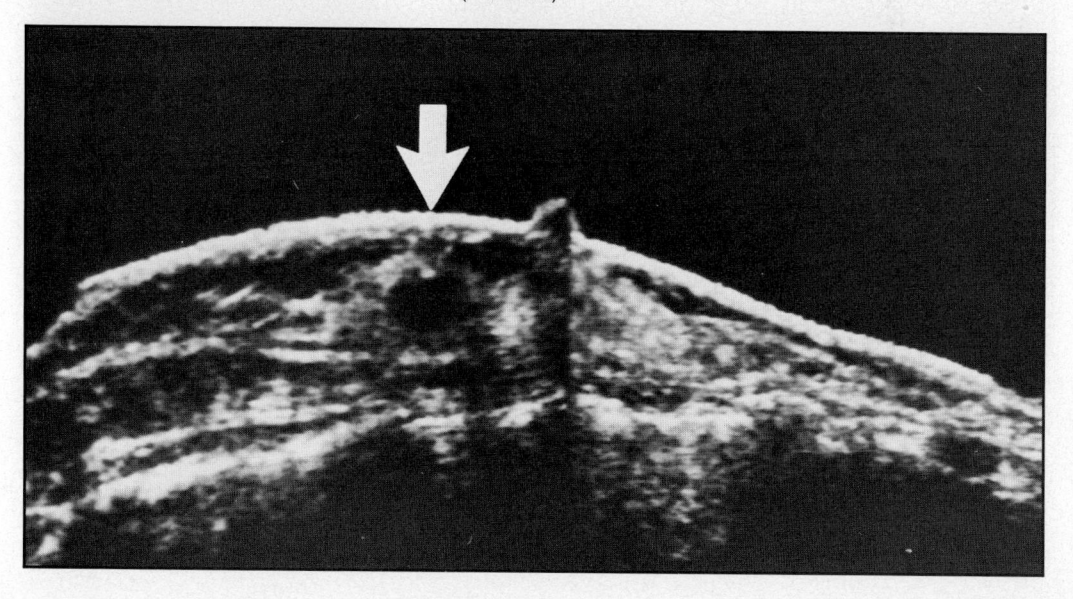

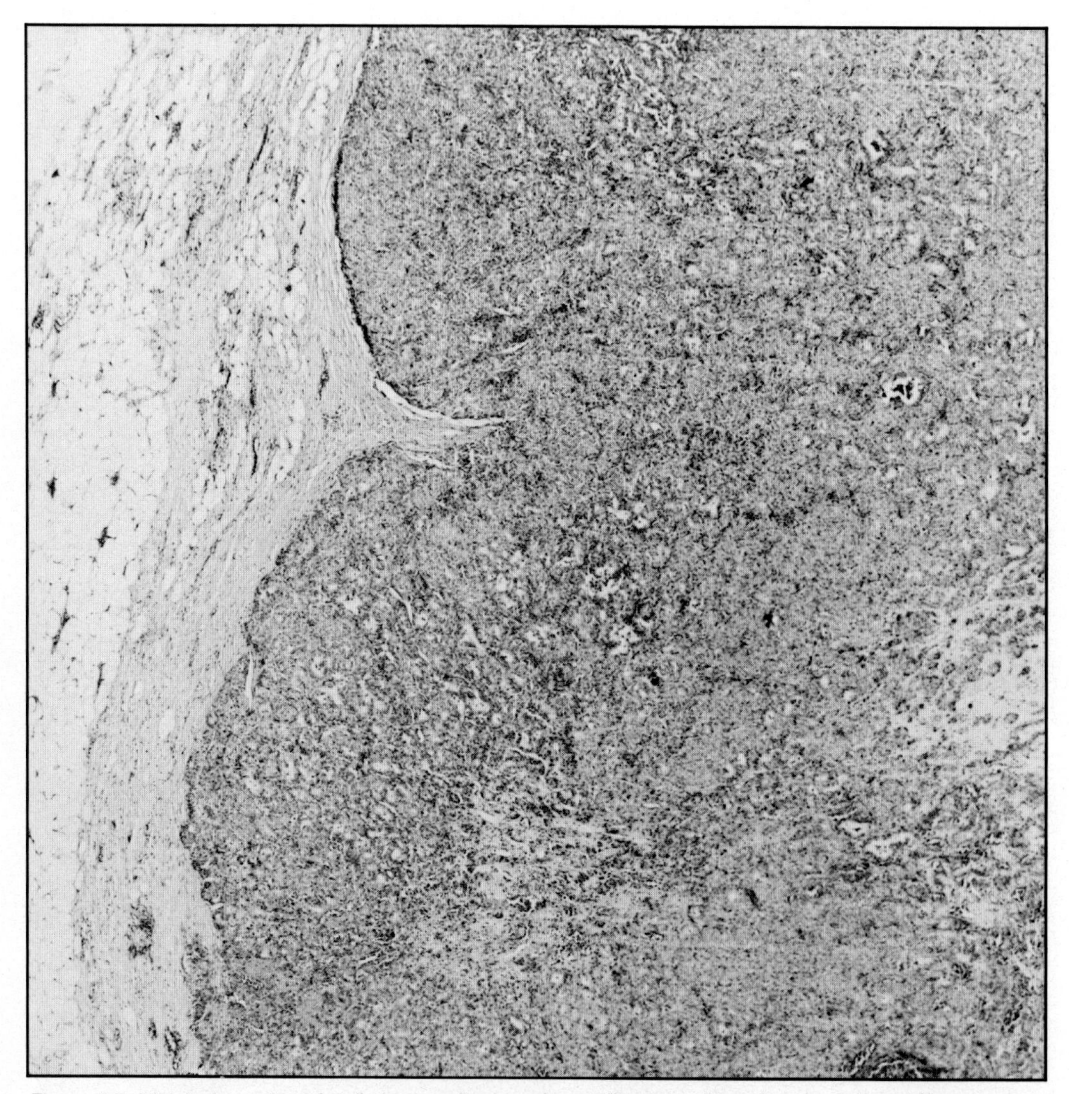

Figure 6-7. Histologic section of well-circumscribed carcinoma (hematoxylin and eosin stain, ×10).

sonographically from benign solid masses. Although ductal carcinomas may occasionally have well-demarcated boundaries (Figure 6-7), most well-circumscribed carcinomas are medullary, papillary, or colloid varieties. The sonographic features of well-circumscribed carcinomas consist of a smooth margin, including anterior and posterior boundaries; moderately strong, homogeneous internal echoes; and variable distal echoes (Figures 6-8 and 6-9).

HISTOLOGIC-SONOGRAPHIC CORRELATION OF BREAST CARCINOMAS

Infiltrating Ductal Carcinoma

This is the most frequently occurring type of breast carcinoma. Grossly, the tumor typically has an irregular margin with stellate strands extending into the surrounding parenchyma (Figure 6-1). In x-ray mammograms the tumor is characteristically dense, with an irregular, spiculated margin, and contains microcalcifications in 40% to 50% of lesions. The ultrasound features are most often those of a poorly-circumscribed carcinoma: ill defined, irregular margins with indistinct posterior boundary, nonuniform low-level internal echoes, and posterior absence of sound or tumor shadowing (Figure 6-2). This shadowing, which may be striking, is believed due to the large proportion of fibrous connective tissue in these tumors.

Lobular Carcinoma

Because this tumor tends not to form a discrete mass, it often goes undetected both in x-ray mammograms and in ultrasonograms (Figure 6-10). Some lobular carcinomas that have been imaged sonographically have shown a fibrous/epithelial ratio and ultrasound features similar to those of infiltrating ductal carcinoma.[3]

Medullary Carcinoma

This uncommon tumor tends to have a more regular margin than infiltrating ductal carcinoma. For this reason, Haagenson prefers to call it "circumscribed carcinoma."[13] On physical examination the tumor is well delimited from the surrounding breast tissue, suggesting benignity. In x-ray mammograms the tumor forms a mass, usually with slightly fuzzy borders but without the spiculation of infiltrating ductal carcinoma, and usually without

118 breast ultrasound

Figure 6-8. Well-circumscribed ductal carcinoma. This 61-year-old woman recently underwent surgery for melanoma of arm. No palpable breast abnormalities.

Figure 6-8A. Mediolateral film-screen mammogram shows relatively well-circumscribed mass.

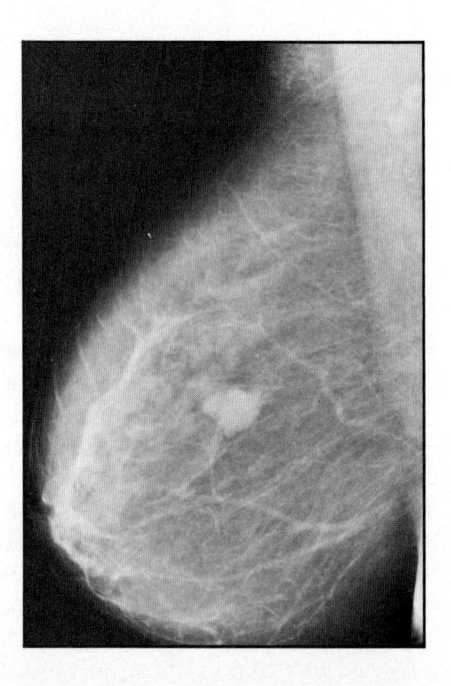

Figure 6-8B. Hand-held real-time examination shows well-circumscribed mass, moderate internal echoes, and lateral edge refraction. These features are usually associated with benign solid masses. Biopsy diagnosis was well-circumscribed ductal carcinoma.

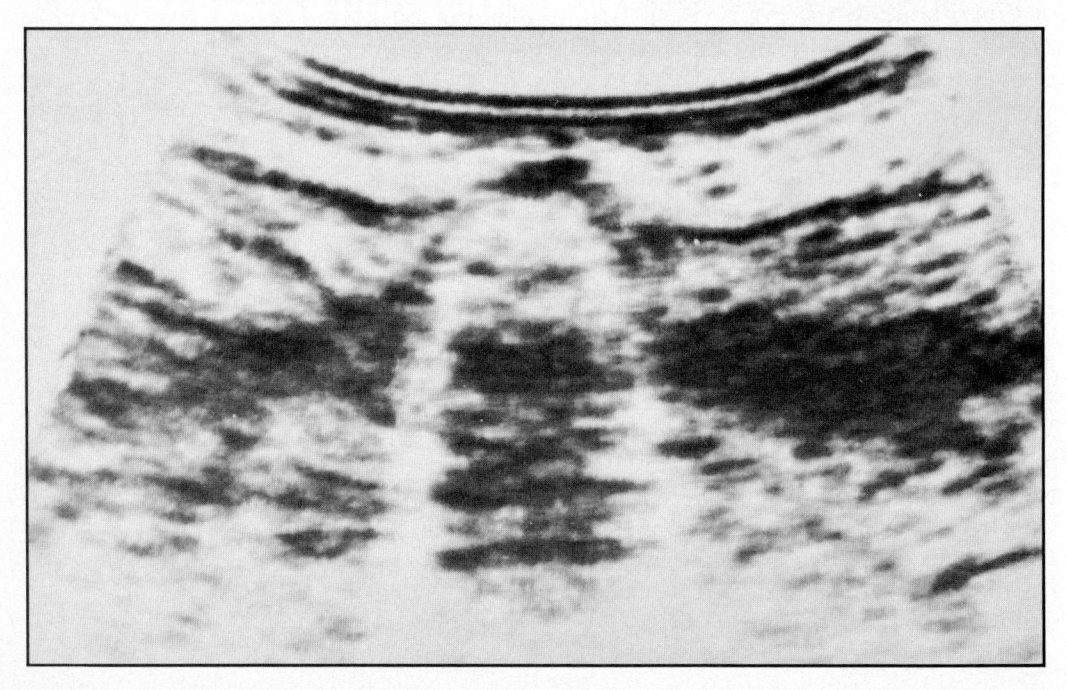

malignant lesions **119**

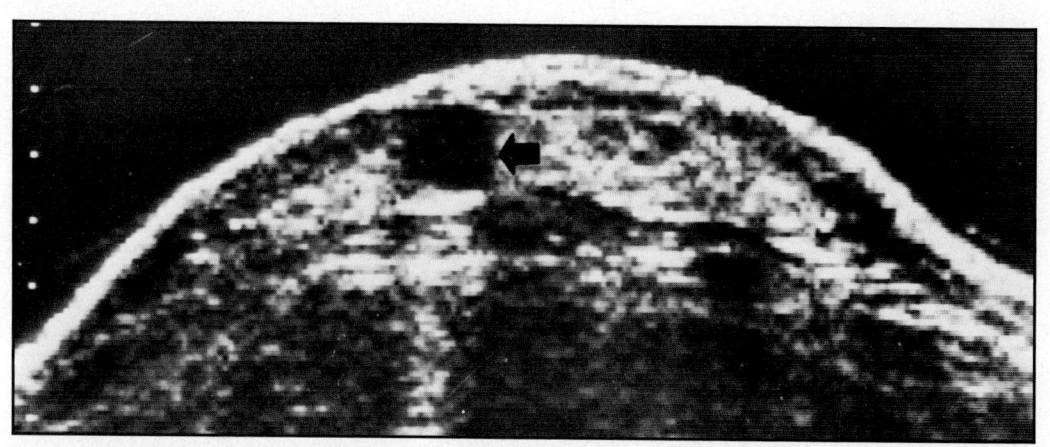

Figure 6-9. Typical medullary carcinoma. Dedicated whole-breast ultrasound, sagittal section. Mass (arrow) is well-defined, internal echoes are weak and irregular. There is distal echo enhancement. (Technicare) Courtesy of Edward A. Sickles, MD, San Francisco, California.

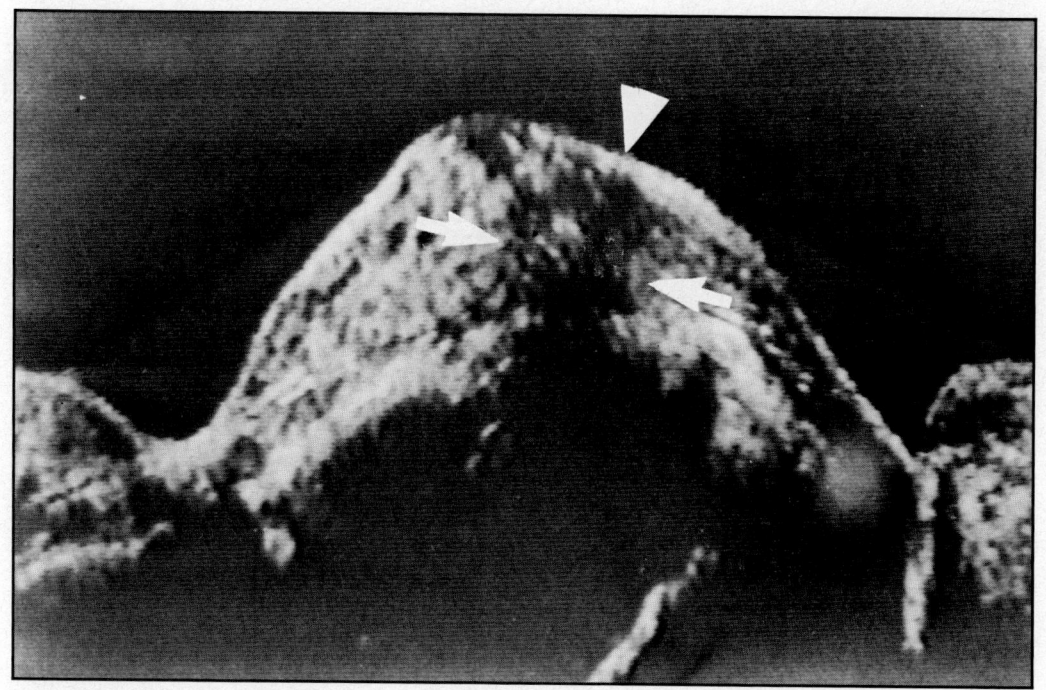

Figure 6-10. Infiltrating lobular carcinoma. Distorted architecture without mass (arrows). There is overlying skin flattening (arrowhead). *From McSweeney: Radiol Cl North Am 23:157, 1985.*

microcalcifications. While its internal echoes are of low intensity and inhomogeneous, they are more numerous than those of infiltrating ductal carcinoma. Because medullary carcinoma is well-circumscibed and contains little if any fibrous connective tissue, it often mimics a benign solid lesion in sonograms (Figure 6-9). Thus, it is characterized by a well-circumscribed margin, low-level homogeneous internal echoes, and a variable effect on posterior echoes. While medullary carcinoma occasionally shows marked distal shadowing, it may alternately display enhanced through-transmission similar to a cyst. Distal shadowing, when present, implies an atypically prominent fibrous connective tissue content.

Papillary Carcinoma

This uncommon type of carcinoma proliferates in a papillary form within ducts and rarely within cysts.[14] It may be difficult to distinguish histologically from a benign papilloma. In x-ray mammograms, papillary carcinoma has a smooth, well-circumscribed margin. Kobayashi[4] reported that the tumor tends toward sonographic features intermediate between poorly circumscribed infiltrating ductal carcinoma and well circumscribed medullary carcinoma (Figure 6-11).

Intracystic papillary carcinoma is rare and tends to occur in older women. On ultrasound it may manifest a mixed cystic and solid echo pattern (Figure 6-12).[15]

Colloid or Mucinous Carcinoma

This tumor is characterized by the presence of mucin secreted by the malignant epithelial cells.[3] Sonographically, through-transmission of sound due to the homogeneous nature of the mucinous material may be sufficiently increased for the tumor to mimic a cyst (Figure 6-13). Aspiration of all presumed solitary cysts is therefore recommended when they are large enough for this to be practical.

malignant lesions **121**

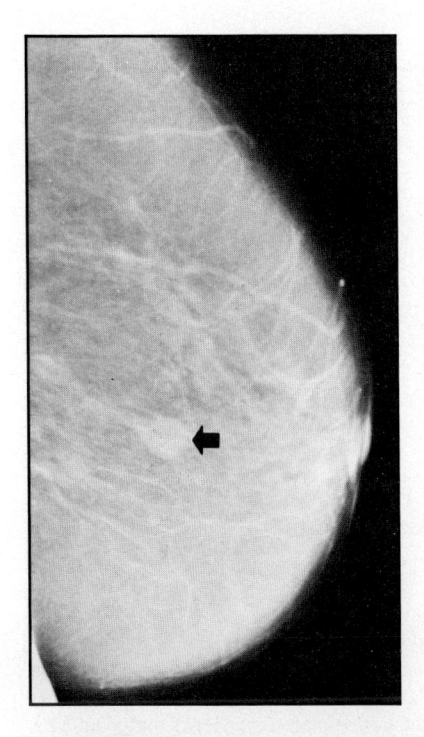

Figure 6-11. Papillary carcinoma. A 58-year-old woman reported palpable mass in left upper outer quadrant. Courtesy of Louise S. O'Shaughnessy, MD, San Diego, California.

Figure 6-11A. Mediolateral mammogram shows 1.5cm mass. Anterior margin is well-circumscribed; however, posterior margin is slightly ill-defined.

Figure 6-11B. Sagittal section of whole-breast ultrasound shows suspicious area of shadowing emanating from the parenchyma. (Technicare)

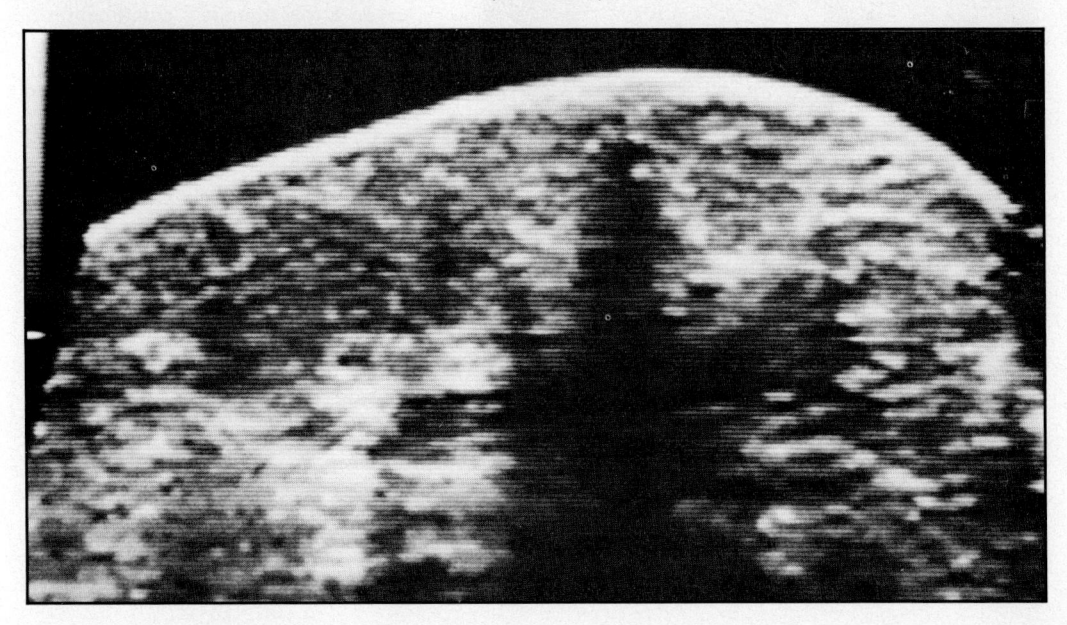

122 breast ultrasound

Figure 6-12. Intracystic papillary carcinoma. *From Reuter: Radiology 153:233, 1984.*

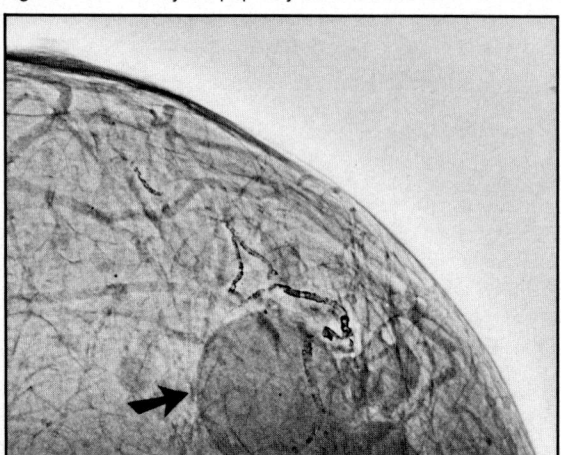

Figure 6-12A. Cephalocaudal xeromammogram shows well-circumscribed masses in left breast. Arrow points to largest mass.

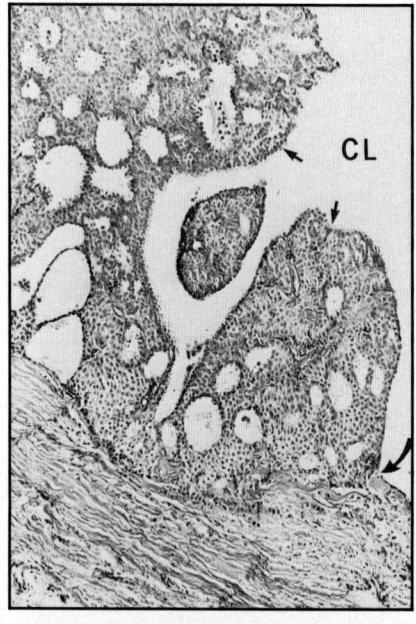

Figure 6-12C. Histologic section. Small arrows show cyst lining composed of malignant cells. Curved arrow identifies demarcation of malignant tumor and benign fibrous tissue.

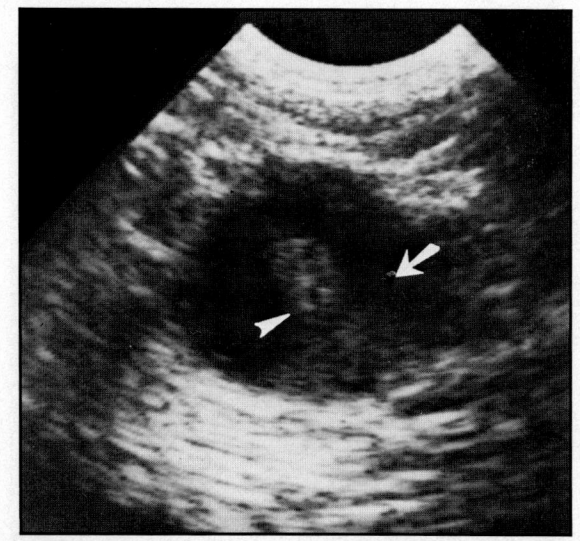

Figure 6-12B. Sonogram shows complex mass of cystic (arrow) and solid components. A solid mass is growing from cyst wall (arrowhead).

malignant lesions **123**

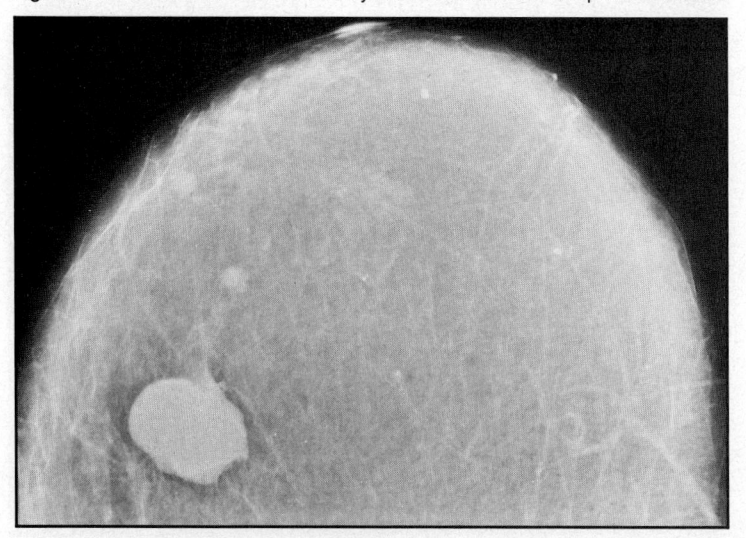

Figure 6-13. Colloid carcinoma. A 73-year-old female with lump in left breast.

Figure 6-13A. Cephalocaudal mammograms reveals fatty breast with one dominant circumscribed mass and several smaller masses.

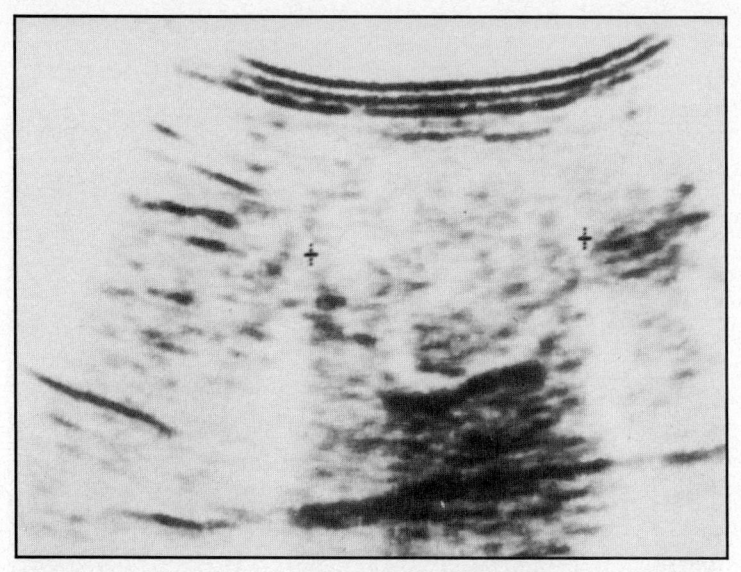

Figure 6-13B. Hand-held ultrasound shows lobulated mass with enhanced posterior echoes. Numerous homogeneous echoes of intensity about equal to surrounding fatty tissue. The tumor would be difficult to identify were it not for the lateral edge refraction shadowing and striking through-transmission.

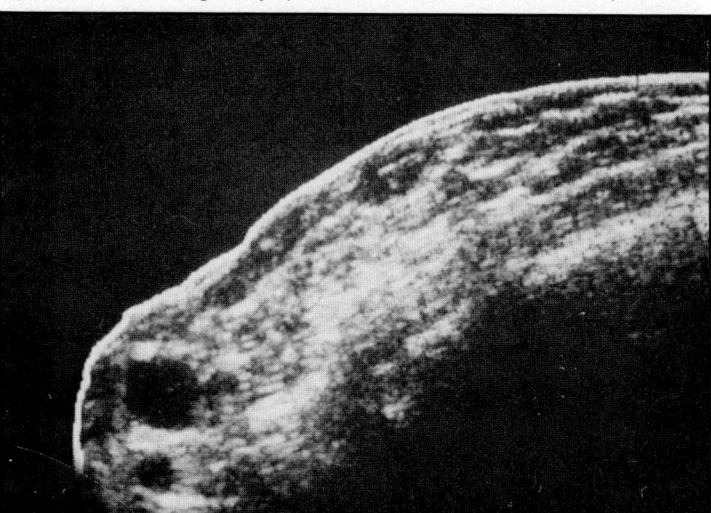

Figure 6-14. Non-Hodgkins lymphoma. *From Derchi: JUM 4:69-74, 1985.*

Figure 6-14A. Two nodules contain a few low-level echoes and yield slight posterior enhancement.

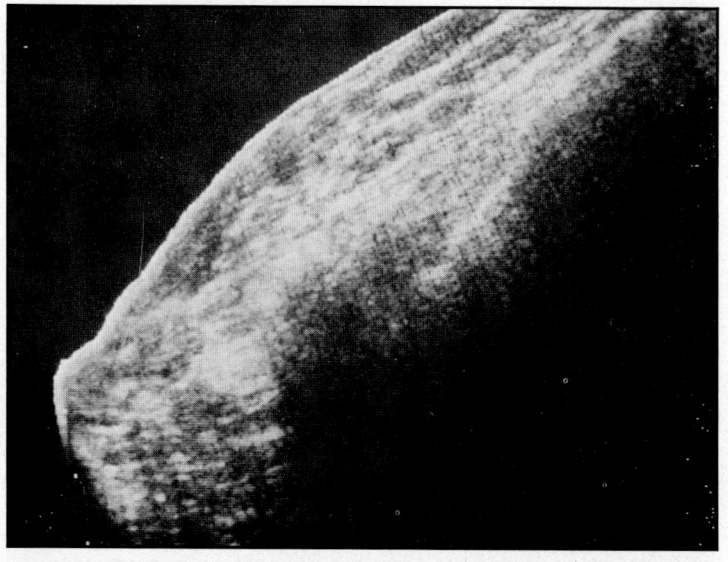

Figure 6-14B. Sonography following chemotherapy shows complete resolution.

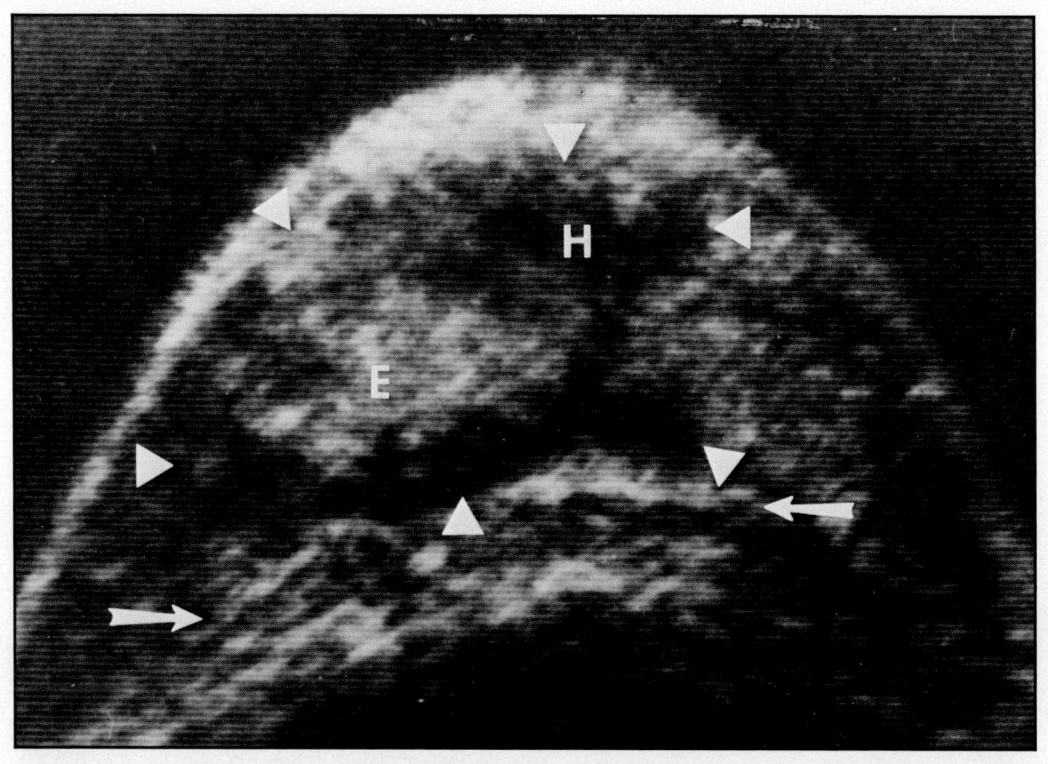

Figure 6-15. Angiosarcoma. A 9cm multilobular mass (arrowheads) contains both highly echoic (E) and hypoechoic (H) areas. Retromammary fascial planes are intact (arrows). *From Grant: AJR 141:691-692, 1983.*

METASTATIC CANCER TO THE BREAST

Metastases to the breast, while uncommon, may originate from almost any extramammary primary malignancy. The metastases may be single or multiple. They tend to be well-circumscribed in mammograms, albeit with a slightly irregular or fuzzy border.[17] Sonographically, breast metastases are usually round or oval with well-defined or slightly irregular borders, manifest a hypoechoic solid internal echo pattern, and have little if any posterior shadowing.[18] Multiple metastatic foci in the same breast tend to have identical sonographic features (Figure 6-14).

SARCOMAS

Sarcomas of the breast are relatively rare. Grant reported the sonographic features of an angiosarcoma.[19] The mass was well-defined and multilobulated with both low- and high-level echoes and no significant attenuation of distal echoes (Figure 6-15).

References

1. Sickles EA, Filly RA, Callen PW: Breast cancer detection with sonography and mammography: Comparison using state-of-the-art equipment. AJR 140:843-845, 1983.
2. Jellins J, Reeve TS, Kossoff G, et al: The ultrasonic characterization of breast malignancies, In Levi S (ed): Ultrasound and Cancer. Amsterdam: Excerpta Medica, 1982, p 283.
3. Cole-Beuglet C, Soriano RZ, Kurtz AB, et al: Ultrasound analysis of 104 primary breast carcinomas classified according to histopathologic type. Radiology 147:191-196, 1983.
4. Kobayashi T, Takatani O, Hattori K: Differential diagnosis of breast tumors. Cancer 33:940-951, 1974.
5. Jellins J, Reeve TS, Kossoff G, et al: The ultrasonic characterization of breast malignancies, In Levi S (ed): Ultrasound and Cancer. Amsterdam: Excerpta Medica, 1983, p 283.
6. Maturo VG, Zusmer NR, Gilson AJ, et al: Ultrasonic appearance of mammary carcinoma with a dedicated whole breast scanner. Radiology 142:713-718, 1982.
7. Teixidor HS, Kazam E: Combined mammographic-sonographic evaluation of breast masses. AJR 128:409-417, 1976.
8. McSweeney MB, Murphy CH: Whole-breast sonography. Radiol Clin North Am 23:157-167, 1985.
9. Kobayashi T: Diagnostic ultrasound in breast cancer: analysis of retrotumorous echo patterns correlated with sonic attenuation by cancerous connective tissue. J Clin Ultrasound 7:471-479, 1979.
10. Egan RL, Egan KL: Automated water-path full-breast sonography: correlation with histology of 176 solid lesions. AJR 143:499-507, 1984.
11. Kopans DB, Meyer JE, Proppe KH: The double line of skin thickening on sonograms of the breast. Radiology 141:485-487, 1981.
12. Kopans DB, Meyer JE, Steinbock RT: Breast cancer: the appearance as delineated by whole breast water-path ultrasound scanning. J Clin Ultrasound 10:313-322, 1982.

13. Haagensen CD: Diseases of the Breast. Philadelphia: W.B. Saunders, 1971, p 570.

14. Haagensen CD: Diseases of the Breast. Philadelphia: W.B. Saunders, 1971, p 528.

15. Reuter K, D'Orsi CJ, Reale F: Intracystic carcinoma of the breast: the role of ultrasonography. Radiology 153:233-234, 1984.

16. Haagensen CD: Diseases of the Breast. Philadelphia: W.B. Saunders, 1971, p 590.

17. Bohman L, Bassett LW, Gold RH, et al: Breast metastases from extramammary malignancies. Radiology 144:309-312, 1982.

18. Derchi LE, Rizzatto G, Giuseppetti GM, et al: Metastatic tumors in the breast: sonographic findings. J Ultrasound Med 4:69-74, 1985.

19. Grant EG, Holt RW, Chun B, et al: Angiosarcoma of the breast: sonographic, xeromammographic, and pathologic appearance. AJR 141:691-692, 1983.

CHAPTER 7

Pitfalls and How to Avoid Them

INTRODUCTION

Diagnostic errors may arise from faulty interpretation or suboptimal performance of breast ultrasound examinations. In addition, there are specific limitations inherent in the various instruments. This chapter reviews some of the more frequent pitfalls and how to avoid them.

PITFALLS IN INTERPRETING THE EXAMINATION

Insufficient Clinical Data

Knowledge of the patient's age, history, physical findings and, when available, x-ray findings are essential when interpreting the examination.[1] For example, in women under 30 years of age, almost all well-circumscribed solid masses are fibroadenomas; however, fibroadenomas are uncommon over age 50, an age group in which well-circumscribed malignancies are more likely to occur. A major pitfall is the performance or interpretation of the examination without knowledge of the location of a palpable or x-ray abnormality. The focus of attention should always be on the clinically suspicious area.

Awareness of the location of a previous surgical or needle aspiration biopsy is essential when interpreting the examination. Biopsy may result in the following findings in the ultrasound examination: asymmetrical acoustic attenuation (either increased or decreased on the side of the biopsy), skin thickening and/or retraction, architectural changes, shadowing, and/or a mass (Figure 7-1). Conservative surgery, lumpectomy or segmentectomy, in combination with radiation therapy is being performed with increasing frequency for the treatment of early breast cancer. Accurate ultrasound evaluation of the treated patient must take into account the resultant changes (Figure 7-2).[2]

Traumatic hemorrhage or fat necrosis may lead to skin thickening or retraction, abnormal sound transmission, or a mass.

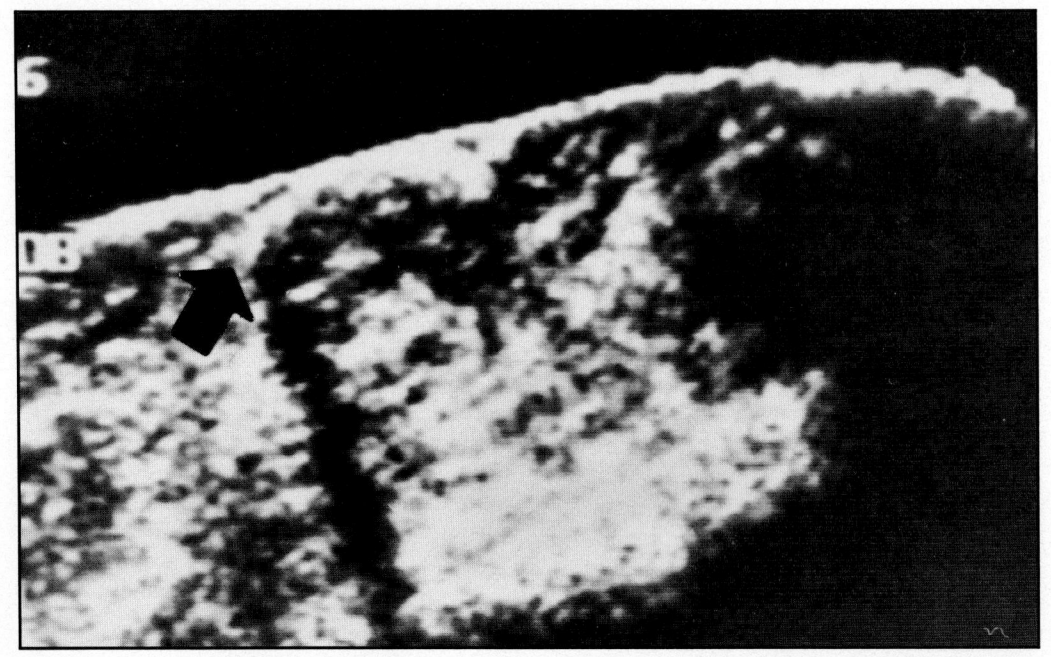

Figure 7-1. Ultrasound one year after breast biopsy. Skin retraction (arrow) and distal shadowing. (Ausonics)

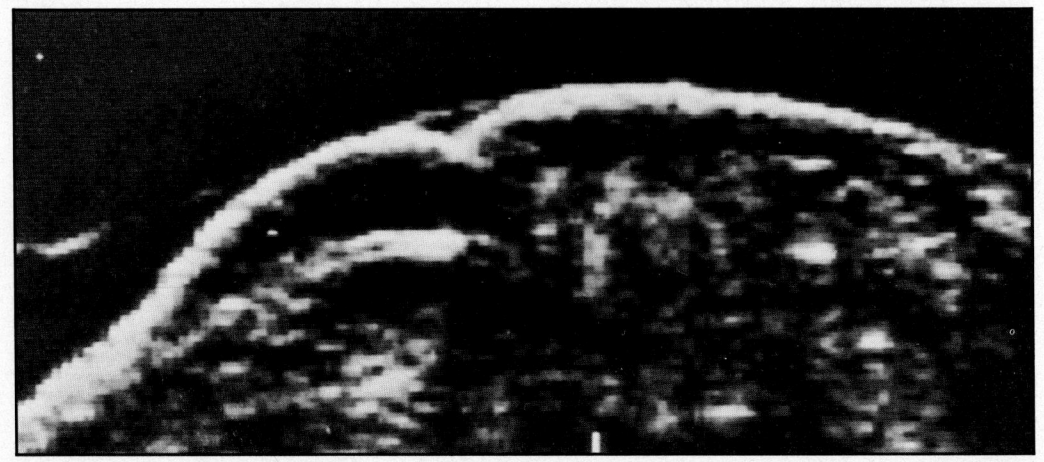

Figure 7-2. Ultrasound examination following lumpectomy and radiation therapy shows skin retraction and diminished echoes at surgical site. (Technicare)

False-Negative Examinations

Sonomammography is not a substitute for x-ray mammography. Ultrasound is particularly limited in the detection of cancer under 1cm, cancer within a fatty breast, and cancers manifested only by microcalcifications in x-ray mammograms.

Failure to Detect Cancer Under 1cm. In one prospective study of 1000 women, ultrasound imaged only 8% of the cancers under 1cm compared to 92% detected by x-ray mammography.[3] Other studies have reported similar results.

Failure to Detect Cancer in Fatty Breasts. Ultrasound frequently fails to demonstrate a cancer in a fatty breast even when obvious on physical examination and in x-ray mammograms (Figure 7-3).[4] Ultrasound images of fatty breasts are generally unsatisfactory because of poor penetration due to reflection and distortion of the beam by multiple interfaces. Despite the low attenuation coefficient of fat, its impedance is so different from that of Cooper's ligaments, ducts, vessels, and parenchymal tissue that the interfaces between these structures and the adjacent fat reflect most of the distorted ultrasound beam back to the transducer.[5] However, x-ray mammography is so highly accurate in fatty breasts that corroborative ultrasound examinations are only rarely indicated.

Failure to Detect Malignant Microcalcifications. X-ray mammograms can depict microcalcifications, frequently the earliest sign of occult malignancy. That microcalcifications are only rarely identified in ultrasound images[6,7,8] is one of the most significant limitations of breast ultrasound.

False-Positive Examinations

Although in breast cancer detection a false-negative examination is more serious than a false-positive one, false-positive examinations result in unnecessary breast biopsies with potential morbidity, possible disfiguration, and added expense.

134 breast ultrasound

Figure 7-3. False-negative ultrasound. A 60-year-old woman felt hard mass 2cm lateral to areola.

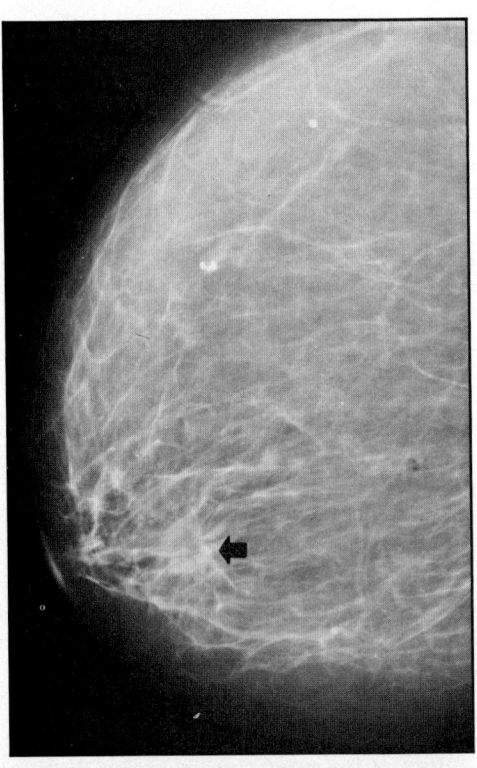

Figure 7-3A. Mediolateral film-screen mammogram. The breast is almost completely fatty. A 2cm spiculated mass (arrow) is present beneath areola.

Figure 7-3B. Automated ultrasound. One of multiple sagittal sections performed in vicinity of mass. There are multiple hypoechoic fat lobules. The cancer was not identified. (Technicare)

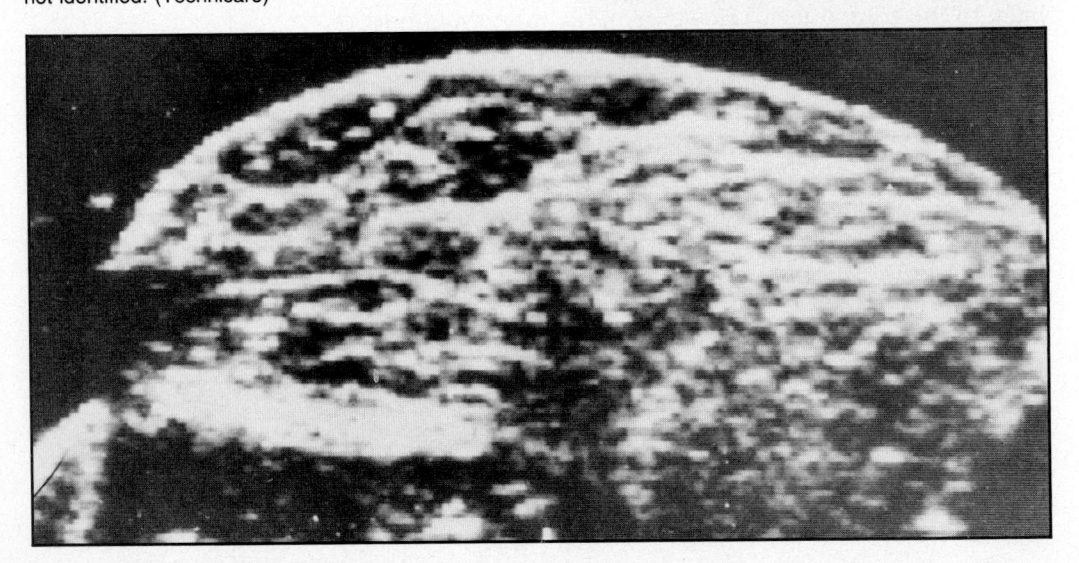

The most common false-positive sonographic "mass" is the fat lobule, particularly the isolated island of fat in a predominantly glandular or fibrous breast. Recognition of the fat lobule depends on carefully following it from one image to the next until all boundaries have been visualized. This will demonstrate that it merges with adjacent fatty tissue. Correlation with the x-ray mammogram is extremely important.

Benign Conditions Presenting with Malignant Features

Benign conditions may occasionally present with what are considered typical malignant ultrasound features: irregular margins and diminished sound transmission distally, secondary signs of malignancy including skin thickening or retraction, and architectural changes. Diminished distal sound transmission, or distal shadowing, is a particularly unreliable indicator of malignancy that may be seen behind a normal nipple, behind Cooper's ligaments, and posterior to any site of increased fibrous tissue proliferation such as a scar or a focus of sclerosing adenosis (Figure 7-4).

PITFALLS IN PERFORMING THE EXAMINATION

In sonomammography a correct diagnosis is dependent on obtaining a technically excellent examination. The breast must be properly positioned for hand-held or automated scanning, and the equipment must be operated in an expert manner. The following examples illustrate pitfalls in the performance of the examination.

Inadequate Penetration of Breast Tissues

Inadequate penetration of specific regions may occur during whole-breast examinations. The center of the breast may be poorly imaged due to nipple shadowing and dense parenchymal tissue. Additional central shadows may arise from connective tissues around the central ducts and from Cooper's ligaments. Methods to improve penetration include

136 breast ultrasound

Figure 7-4. Benign condition presenting with malignant features. A 40-year-old woman felt left breast mass.

Figure 7-4A. Mediolateral x-ray mammogram shows large, well-circumscribed mass.

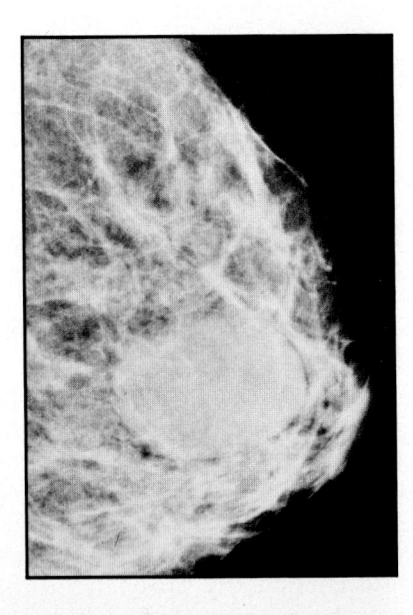

Figure 7-4B. Whole-breast ultrasound, sagittal section, reveals hypoechoic mass with distal shadowing. Ultrasound diagnosis was carcinoma. Biopsy revealed focus of sclerosing adenosis.

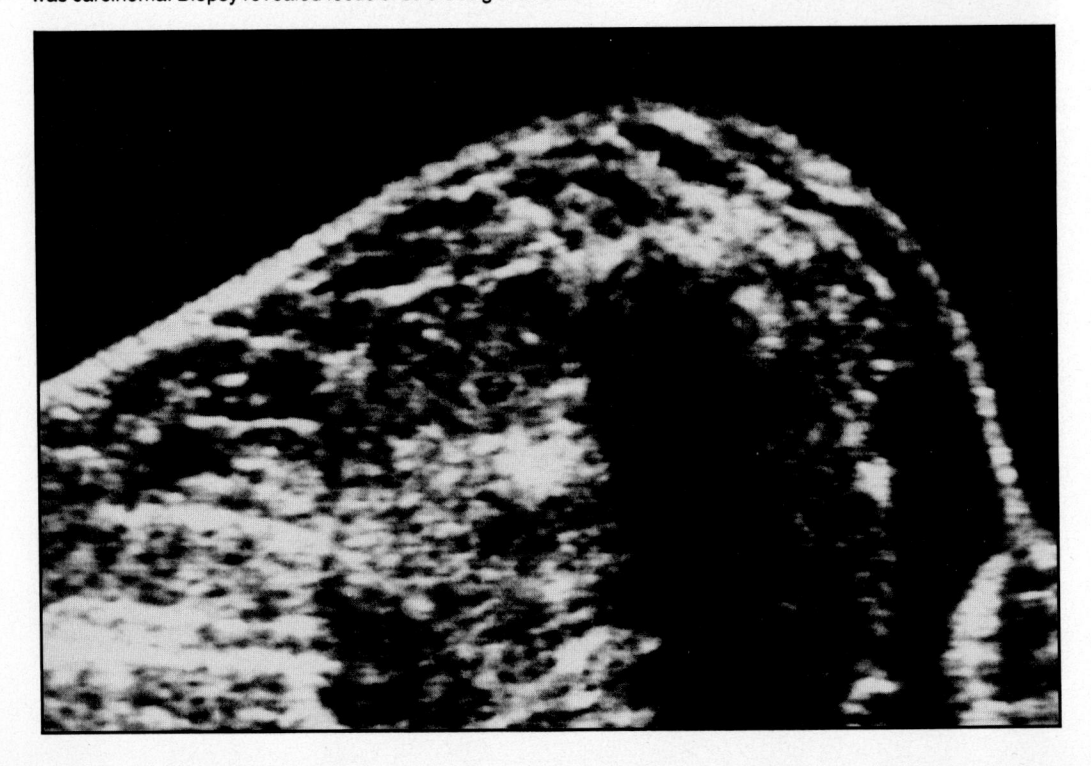

the use of greater power, different transducers, and/or breast compression (Figure 7-5).

Inadequate acoustic penetration of the lateral and medial aspects of the breast may occur in water-path examinations when the patient is prone and the breast is compressed with a plastic sheet. This is due to critical angle refraction at the curved skin or fat/glandular tissue interface at the medial and lateral breast surfaces (Figure 7-6). This problem can be solved only by repositioning the patient and the breast in order to perform additional scans with the appropriate areas centered over the transducer. For example, to image the lateral tissues, the patient should be turned so that the outer part of her breast is over the center of the tank, following which compression is applied again.

Imaging Cysts and Anechoic Masses

With the application of excessive power, echoes can be produced in cysts and other anechoic masses. These "artifactual" echoes will be restricted to the anterior portions of the interior of the mass. In contrast, a solid mass will have echoes throughout its interior.

Debris within a fluid-filled cyst will also produce internal echoes. However, repositioning the patient will usually cause a shift in the location of the debris to the most dependent portion of the cyst.

Masses Near the Chest Wall

When a mass is adjacent to the chest wall, distal acoustic enhancement or shadowing may be diminished due to sound attenuation by the dense chest wall structures. In order to show acoustic effects in the posterior-most breast tissue during a hand-held real-time examination, the patient should be repositioned so that she is nearly prone. The transducer beam should then be directed from the side. This may permit the imaging of the posterior wall of the mass, which has now become dependent, as well as some breast tissue behind it.

The Male Breast

Ultrasound mammography is useful to evaluate male

138 breast ultrasound

Figure 7-5. Inadequate penetration of breast.

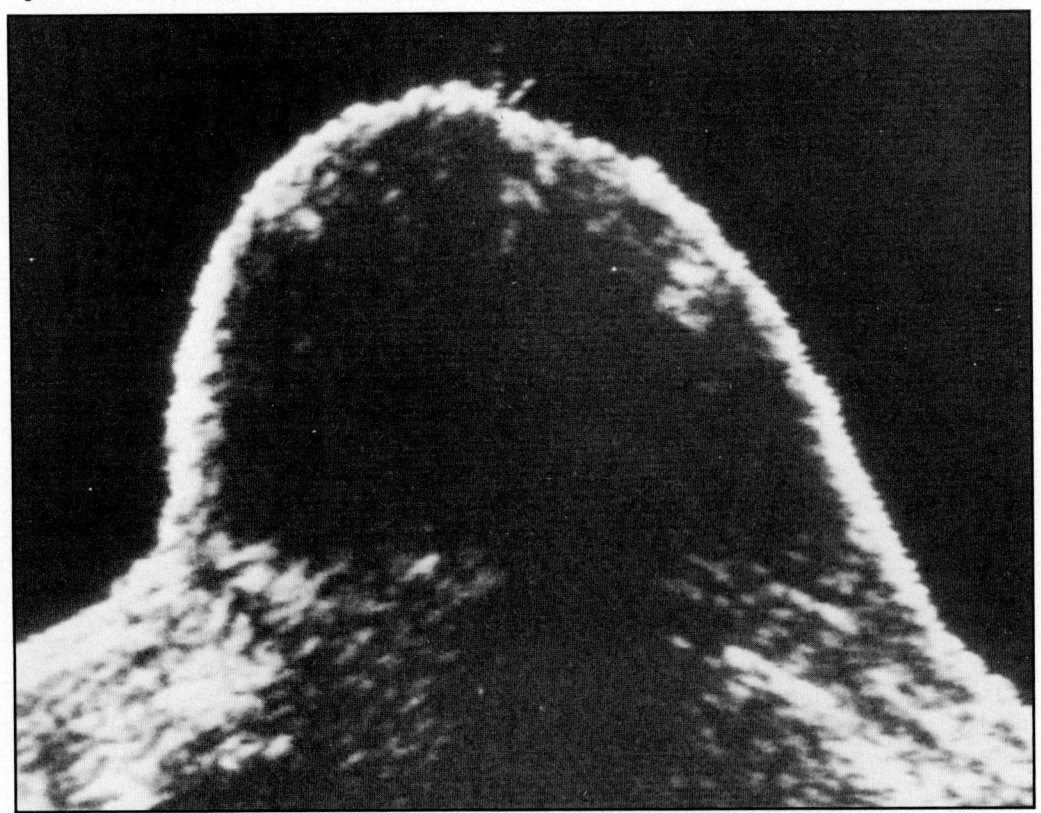

Figure 7-5A. Noncompressed (free-hanging).

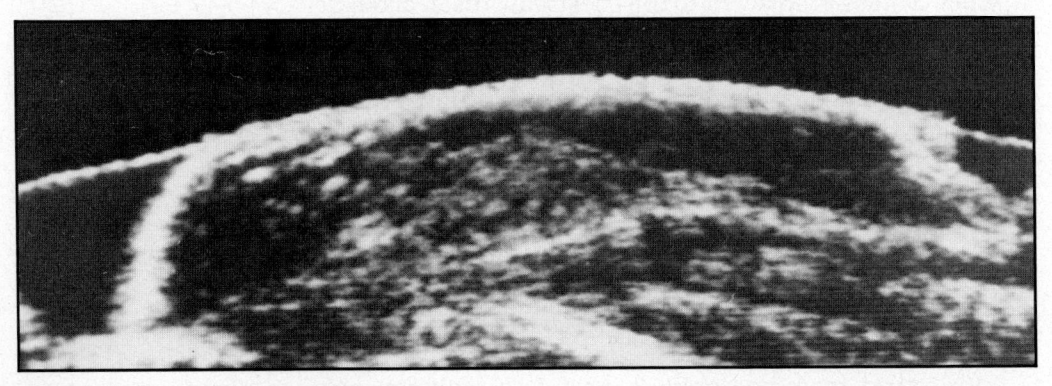

Figure 7-5B. Compression.

pitfalls **139**

Figure 7-6. Poor penetration due to critical angle refraction.

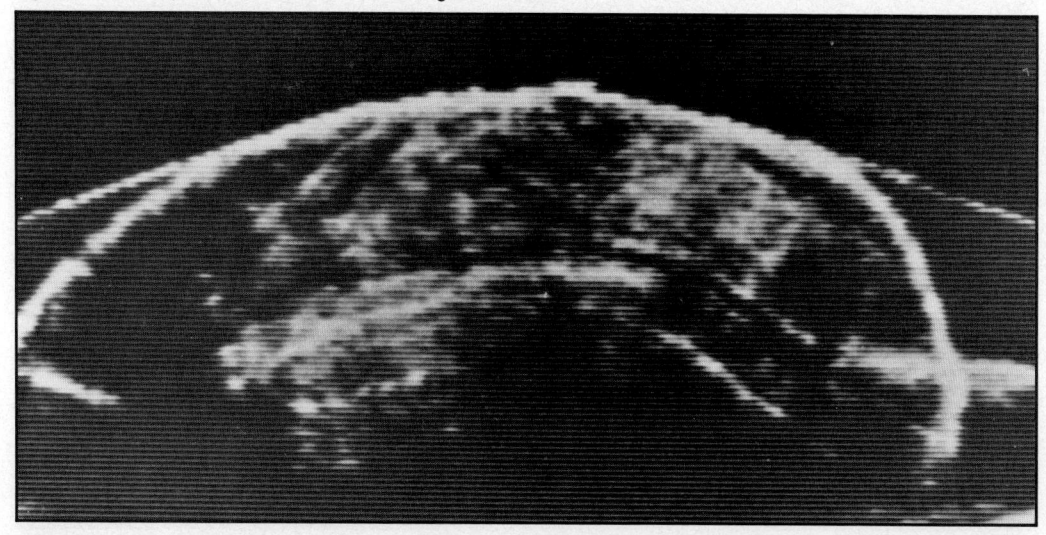

Figure 7-6A. Poor penetration of lateral aspects of compressed breast in water-path may be due to critical angle refraction.

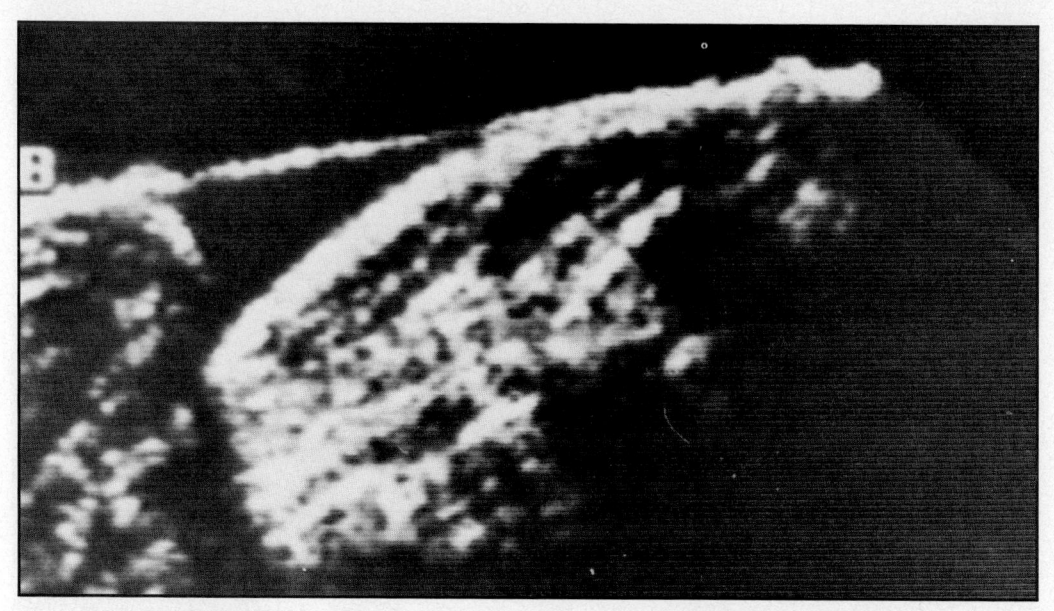

Figure 7-6B. Adequate penetration of lateral aspect is achieved by re-positioning the lateral portion of breast more directly over water tank.

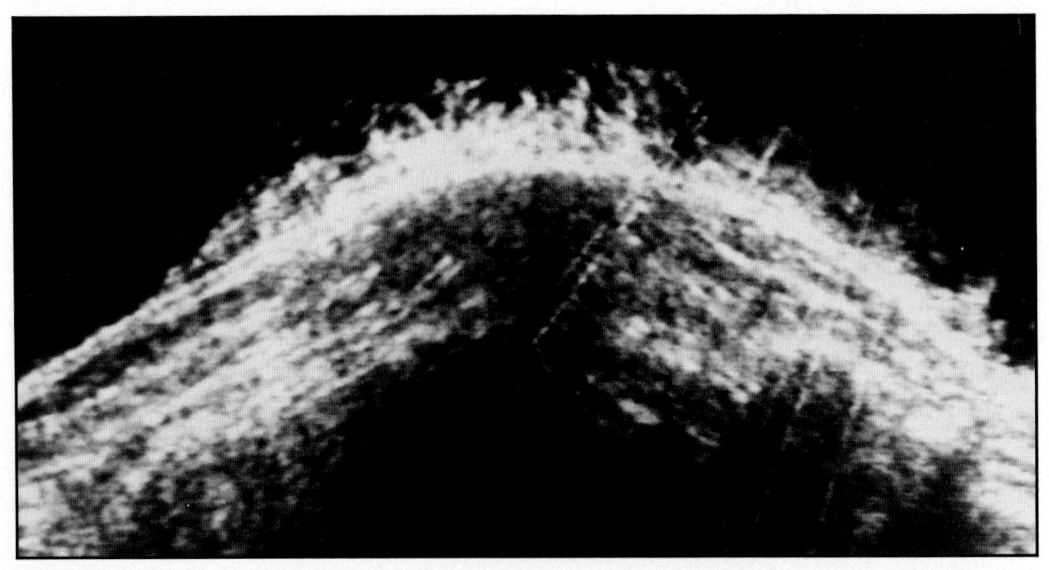

Figure 7-7. Male breast examination. Hair on chest pretriggers TGC and disrupts beam.

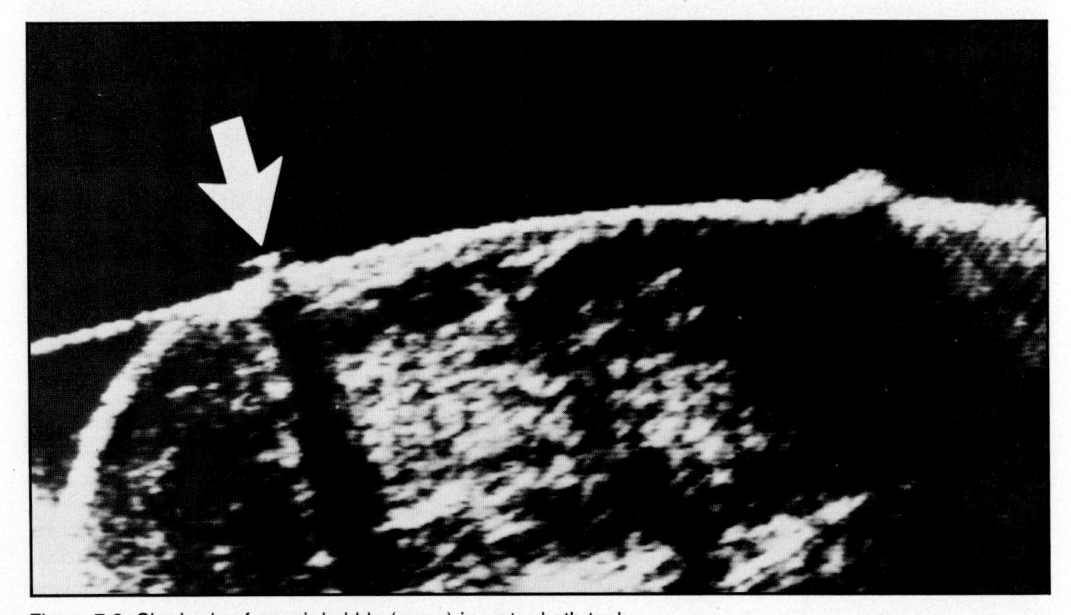

Figure 7-8. Shadowing from air bubble (arrow) in water-bath tank.

breast enlargment or masses.[9] Because hair on the chest may disrupt the beam pattern and degrade the image (Figure 7-7), shaving the area prior to scanning is recommended.

Instrument-Dependent Pitfalls

Different types of real-time or automated ultrasound equipment may produce vastly different images of the same breast. Furthermore, the same unit operated by different technologists may give varying images. There are inherent advantages and limitations to specific types of equipment. It is important to learn the characteristics of the instrument you are using and how to use it optimally. Certain artifacts may be limited to specific scanning methods or instruments (Figure 7-8).

Here are examples of how the operator can alter the focal zone of different instruments in order to determine whether a mass detected by palpation or in an x-ray mammogram is cystic or solid:

Hand-Held Real-Time Examination. If the mass is in the near field of the transducer, an alternate transducer with a different focal zone should be tried. If additional transducers are not available, a water bag spacer should be applied to bring the mass into the focal zone of the transducer.

Automated Whole-Breast Examination. Correct focal zone placement is achieved in a different way with each unit. Using the Technicare unit, the technologist should image the mass entirely above or below the field mark. The focal zone of the Ausonics unit should optimally be placed in the lower half of the mass and a single transducer should be used. With the Labsonics unit, the operator should avoid imaging the mass in the near zone.

References

1. Cole-Beuglet CC, Kurtz AB, Rubin CS, Goldberg BB: Ultrasound mammography. Radiol Clin North Am 18:133-143, 1980.

2. Grant EG, Richardson JD, Citgay OS, et al: Sonography of the breast: findings following conservative surgery and irradiation for early carcinoma. Radiology 147:535-539, 1983.

3. Sickles EA, Filly RA, Callen PW: Breast cancer detection with sonography and mammography: comparison using state-of-the-art equipment. AJR 140:843-845, 1983.

4. Croll J: Ultrasonic diagnosis of malignant tumors of the breast, *In* Kossoff G, Fukuda M (eds): Ultrasonic Differential Diagnosis of Tumors. New York: Igaku-Shoin, 1984, p 90.

5. Davros WJ, Madsen EL, Zagzebski JA: Breast mass detection by US: a phantom study. Radiology 156:773-775, 1985.

6. Egan RL, Egan KL: Automated water-path full-breast sonogaphy: Correlation with histology of 176 solid lesions. AJR 143:499-507, 1984.

7. Lambie RW, Hadgden D, Herman EM, et al: Sonomammographic manifestations of mammographically detectable breast microcalcifications. J Ultrasound Med 509-514, 1983.

8. Perez-Mendez V, Wiedenbeck P, Danis P, et al: Ultrasound imaging and identification of microcalcifications and clusters by correlation of scatter from multiple angles. IEEE Trans Med Imag MI-3:124-130, 1984.

9. Cole-Beuglet C, Schwartz GF, Kurtz AB, et al: Ultrasound mammography for male breast enlargement. J Ultrasound Med 1:301-306, 1982.

CHAPTER 8

Quiz Cases

Introduction

The following quiz cases will help to reinforce the information and concepts presented in the previous chapters. The discussion of each case is divided into three parts: problem, image analysis, and solution. For each case, analyze the images, and make a diagnosis and/or recommend further diagnostic workup.

Problem 1:

A 43-year-old woman noted a soft palpable mass in her left breast. Needle aspiration of the mass yielded clear fluid, but at the time of aspiration another mass was palpated in the same breast. Bilateral mammograms revealed only dense parenchymal tissue. Two transverse sections from an automated ultrasound examination are shown in Figure 8-1A.

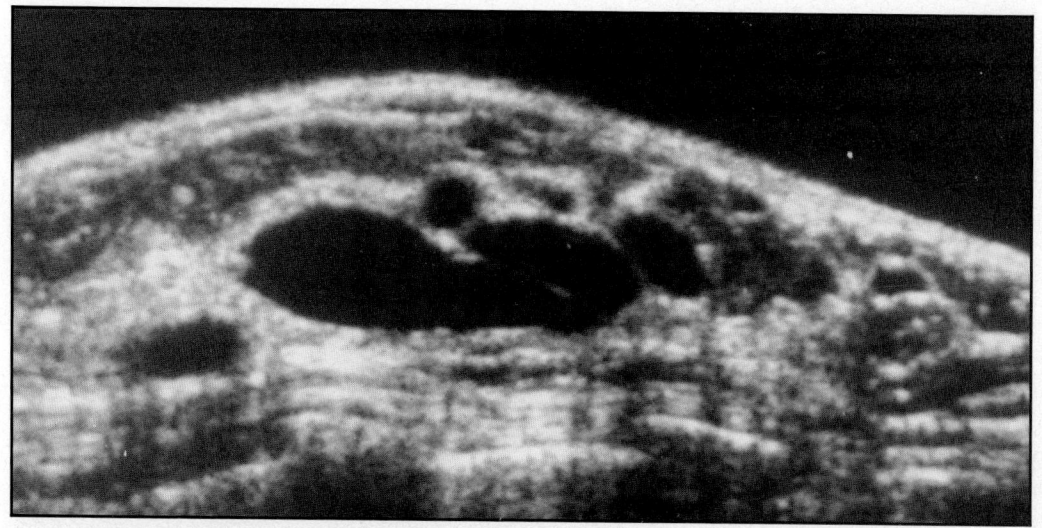

Figure 8-1A. Transverse section from automated ultrasound. (Labsonics)

148 breast ultrasound

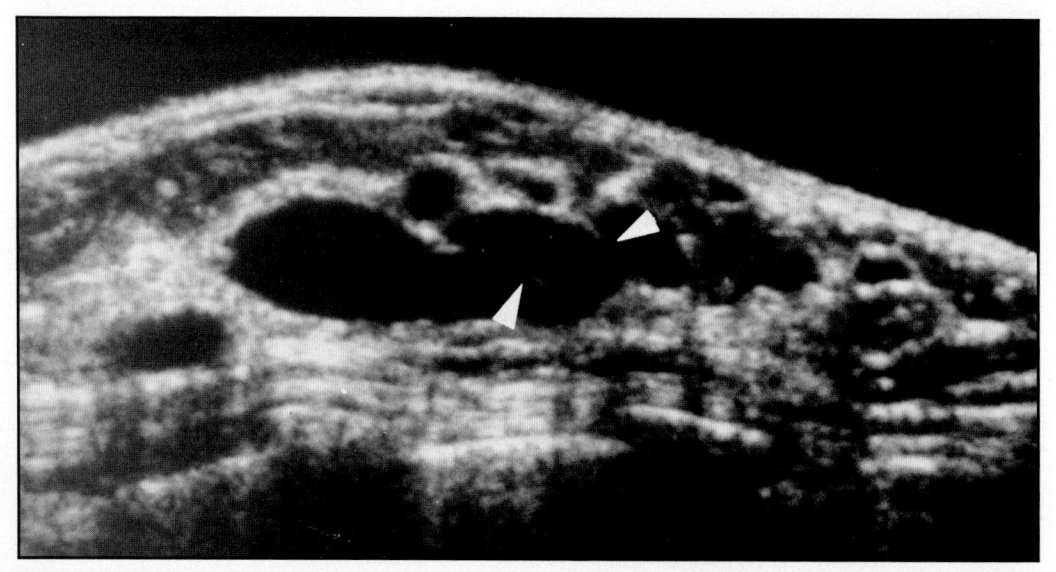

Figure 8-1B. Multiple well-marginated anechoic masses have weak-to-moderate enhancement of echoes distally. There are several linear structures within the largest mass (arrowheads). (Courtesy of Joel Sokoloff, MD, Poway, California.)

Solution:

Multiple well-circumscribed anechoic masses with weak-to-moderate enhancement of echoes distally are features characteristic of cysts. The largest cyst contains several septae (arrowheads). No further diagnostic workup is needed. (Courtesy of Joel Sokoloff, MD, Poway, California.)

Problem 2:

A 43-year-old woman had a 1.5cm mass in the upper hemisphere of her right breast. She had had three previous biopsies of fibroadenomas. X-ray mammography and hand-held ultrasonography were performed.

quiz cases 151

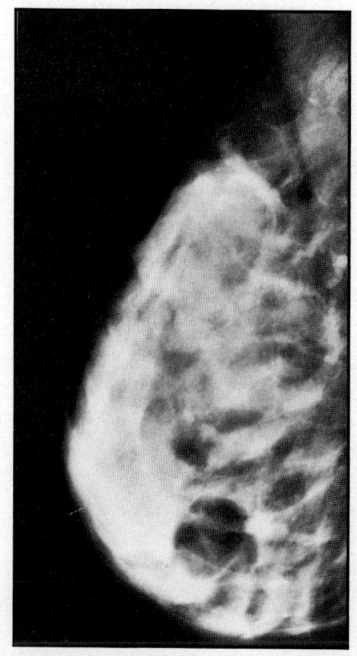

Figure 8-2A. Oblique x-ray mammogram of right breast.

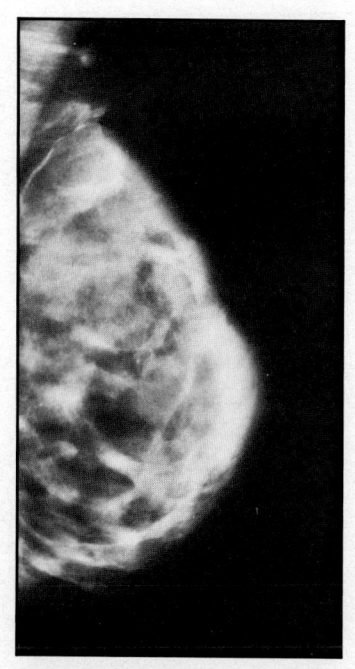

Figure 8-2B. Oblique x-ray mammogram of left breast.

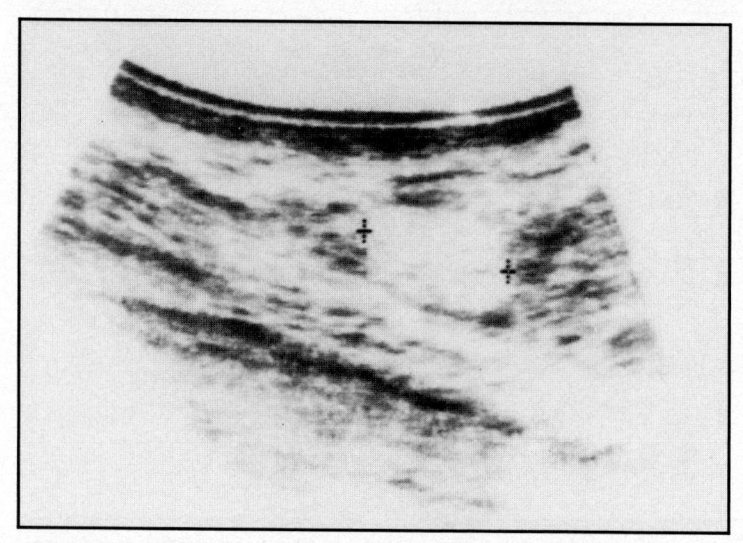

Figure 8-2C. Hand-held real-time ultrasound image of upper hemisphere of right breast.

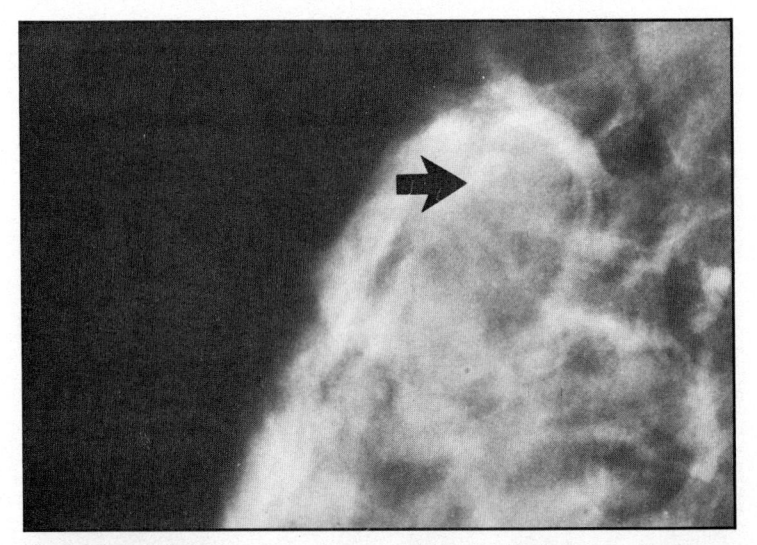

Figure 8-2D. Oblique x-ray mammogram, right breast. Well-circumscribed mass is present superiorly (arrow). We noted mass only in retrospect, after performing sonography.

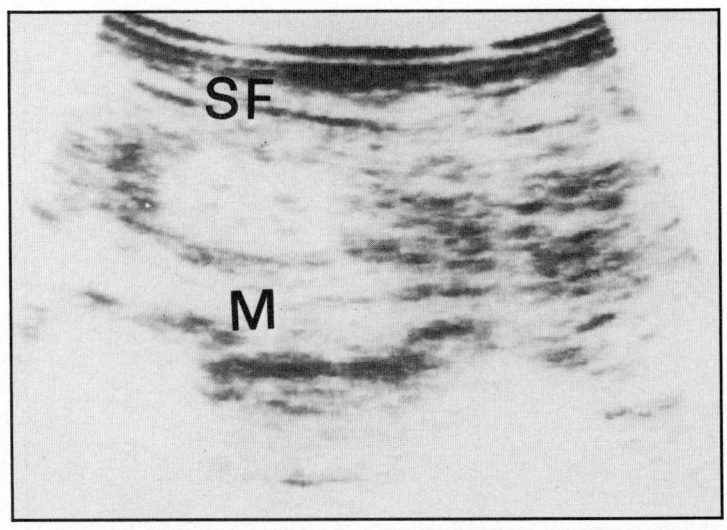

Figure 8-2E. Hand-held real-time ultrasound shows well-defined mass lying between subcutaneous fat (SF) and pectoral muscle (M).

Solution:

Because of the generalized increase in parenchymal density, a well-circumscribed 1.5cm mass was noted only retrospectively in the upper hemisphere of the right breast (Figure 8-2D), after ultrasound showed a well-circumscribed mass with low-level echoes, suggesting fibroadenoma (Figure 8-2E). Biopsy confirmed fibroadenoma.

Problem 3:

A 48-year-old woman with no breast complaints was referred for routine x-ray mammograms. An abnormality was observed on one of the mammograms. Ultrasound was performed.

quiz cases 155

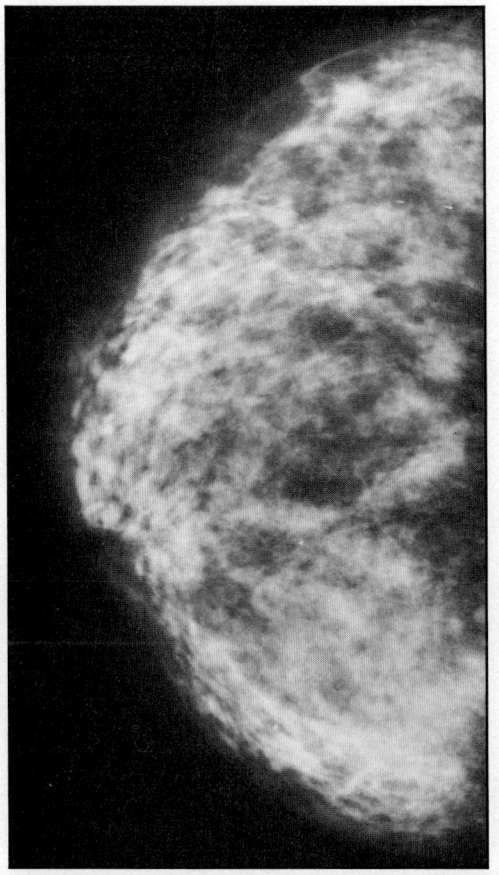

Figure 8-3A. Right mediolateral x-ray mammogram.

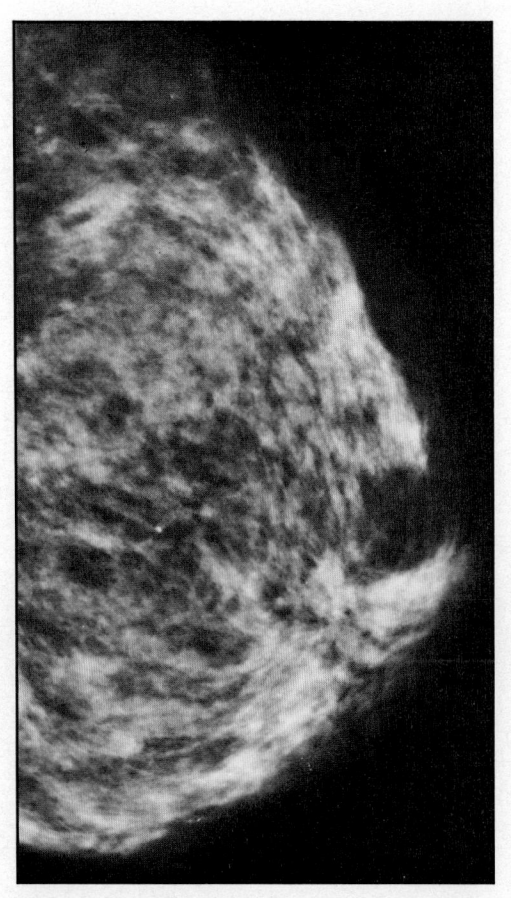

Figure 8-3B. Left mediolateral x-ray mammogram.

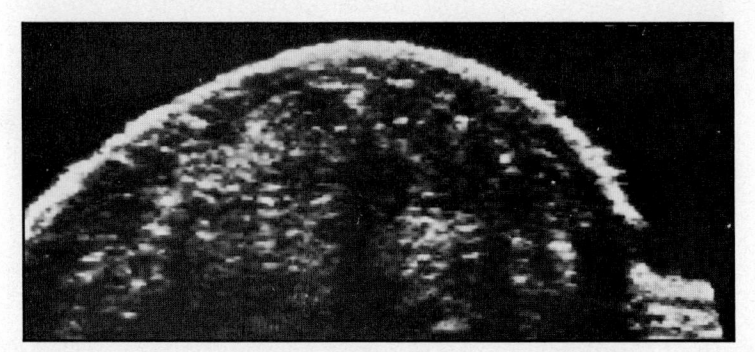

Figure 8-3C. Dedicated ultrasound, longitudinal section. (Technicare)

156   breast ultrasound

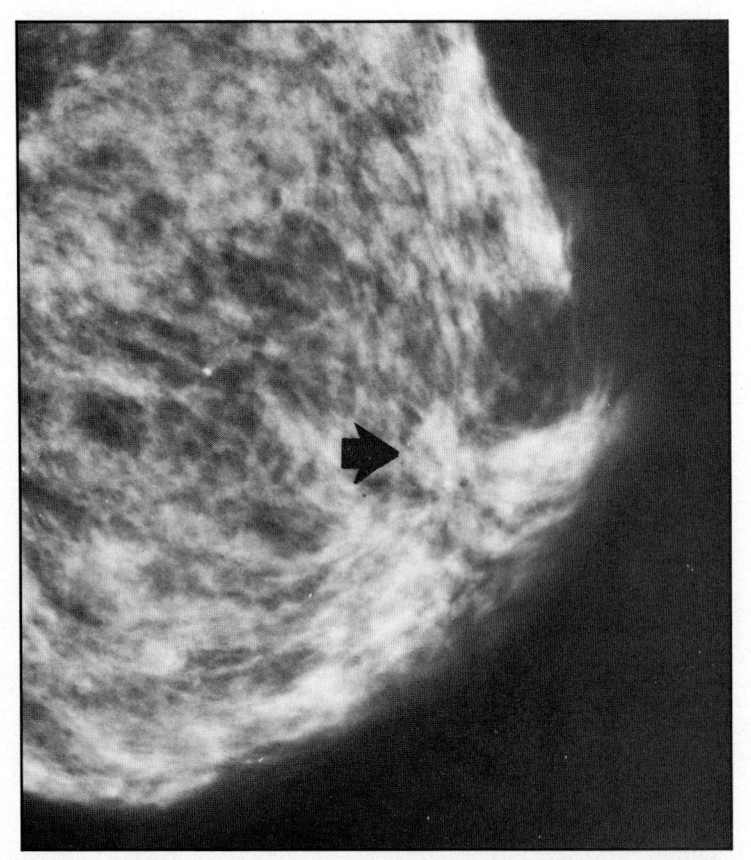

Figure 8-3D. Mediolateral x-ray mammogram of left breast discloses 1.5cm mass with irregular border (arrow).

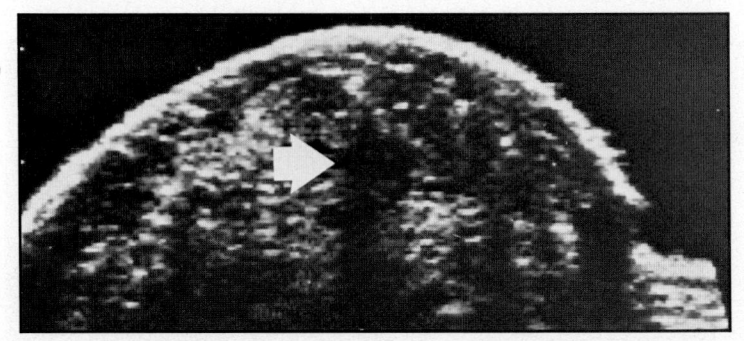

Figure 8-3E. Dedicated ultrasound. Mass (arrow) has irregular margin, is hypoechoic, and produces distal shadowing.

Solution:

The x-ray mammograms feature a bilaterally prominent duct pattern. A 1.5cm mass with an irregular margin is present 2cm deep to the nipple in the mediolateral view of the left breast (Figure 8-3D). Automated ultrasound confirms the presence of the mass and localizes it to a site 1cm medial to the nipple (Figure 8-3E). The mass results in considerable distal echo attenuation. The findings in x-ray and ultrasound studies are characteristic of carcinoma. Biopsy revealed infiltrating carcinoma.

Problem 4:

A 49-year-old woman complained of a rapidly growing mass in the left breast for one month. X-ray mammogram and hand-held real-time ultrasound images of the breast are presented in Figure 8-4.

quiz cases 159

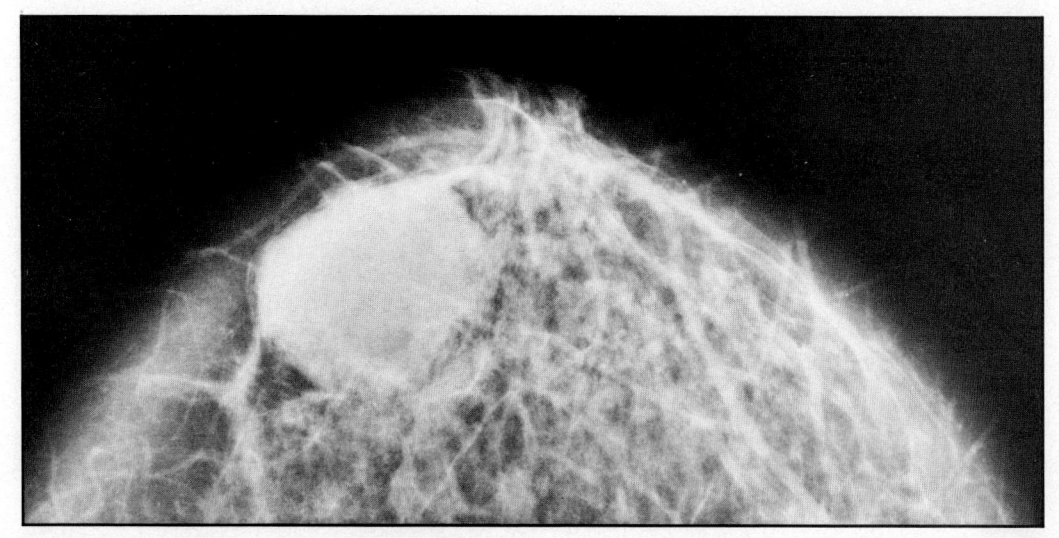

Figure 8-4A. Cephalocaudal x-ray mammogram.

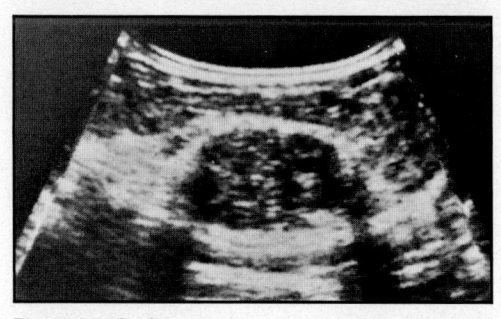

Figure 8-4B. Section from hand-held ultrasound examination.

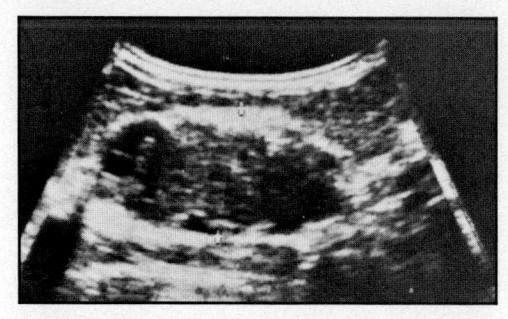

Figure 8-4C. Section from hand-held ultrasound examination.

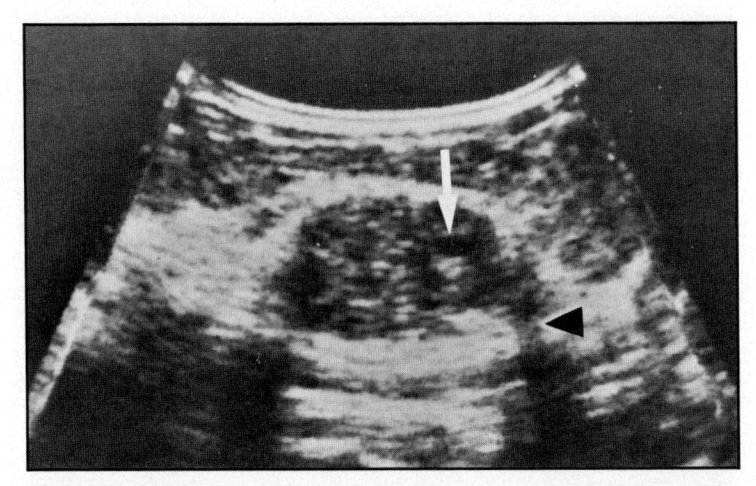

Figure 8-4D. Ultrasound reveals a well-delineated solid mass with a thick capsule. The mass manifests cystic foci (arrow) and lateral edge refraction (arrowhead).

Solution:

In the x-ray mammogram, the homogeneous breast mass has a smooth margin, except posteriorly. The posterior indistinctness of the border of an otherwise smoothly marginated mass should suggest the possibility of a well-circumscribed carcinoma. The ultrasound image proves that the mass is basically solid but contains a combination of hyperechoic, hypoechoic, and anechoic regions (Figure 8-4D). The mixture of solid (echoic) and cystic (anechoic) features is reportedly characteristic of cystosarcoma. Although the ultrasound features of a well-circumscribed margin and lateral refraction suggest a benign mass, in this age group a well-circumscribed malignancy is just as likely. Biopsy revealed benign cystosarcoma phylloides.

Problem 5:
A 46-year-old woman complained of breast lumps. In the past, she had multiple cyst aspirations. X-ray mammography and ultrasonography were performed (Figure 8-5).

quiz cases   **163**

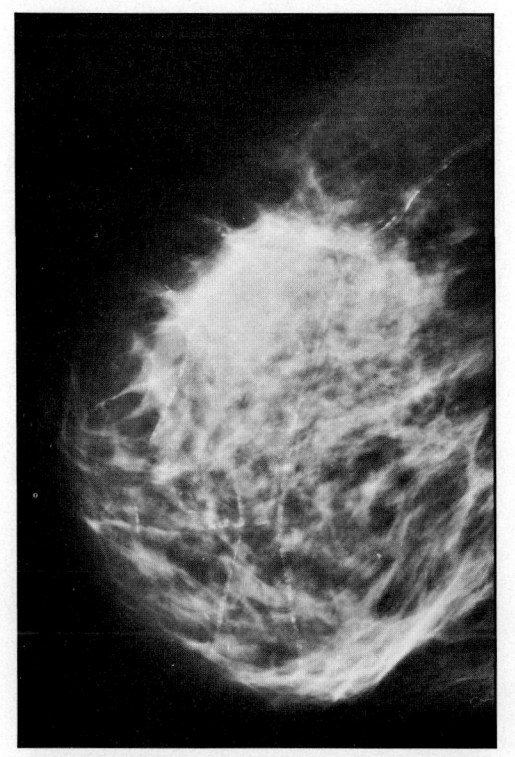

Figure 8-5A. Right mediolateral x-ray mammogram.

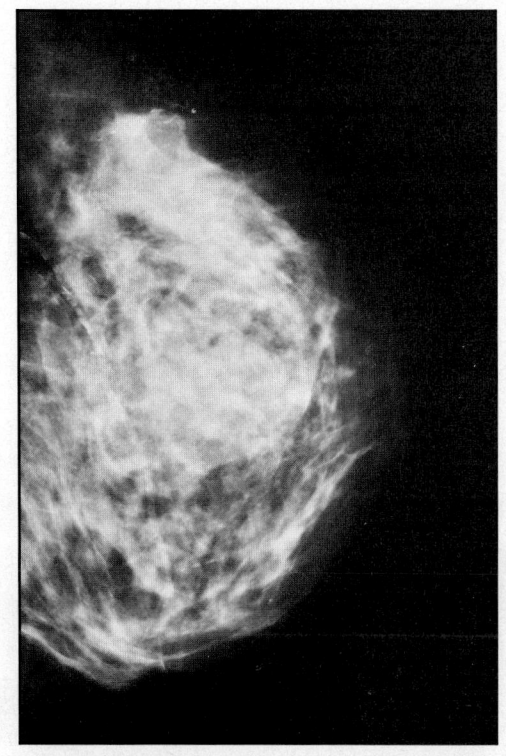

Figure 8-5B. Left mediolateral x-ray mammogram.

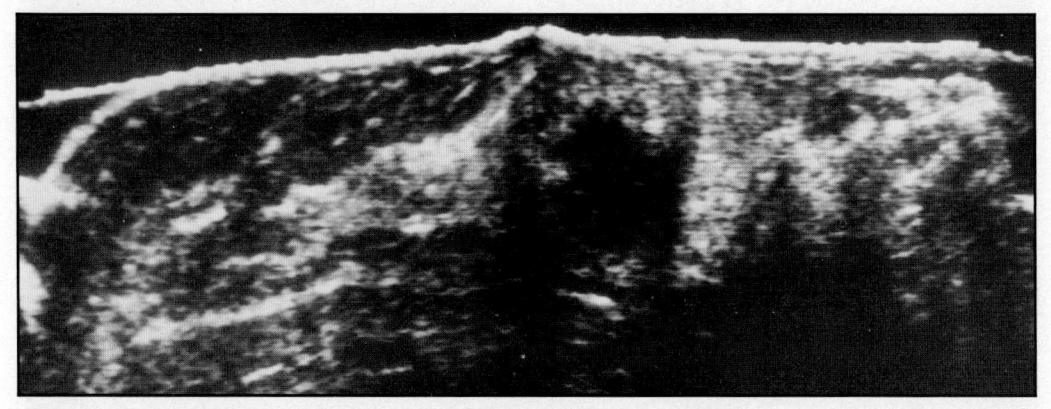

Figure 8-5C. Longitudinal section from left automated whole-breast ultrasound examination performed with compression. (Ausonics)

164 breast ultrasound

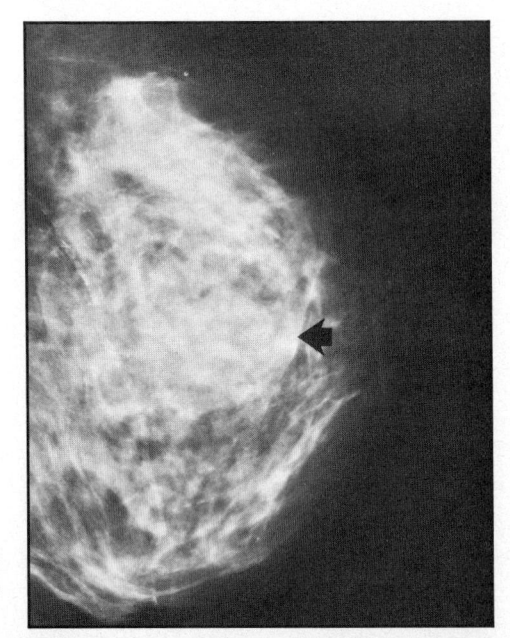

Figure 8-5D. Arrow indicates ill-defined, bilaterally asymmetric, subareolar density in x-ray mammogram of left breast.

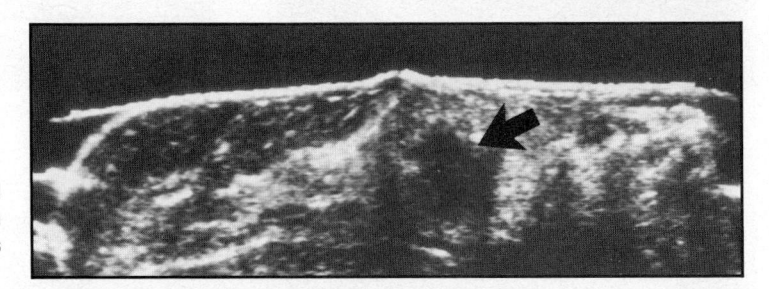

Figure 8-5E. Automated ultrasound image showed an irregular hypoechoic mass (arrow) deep to the nipple.

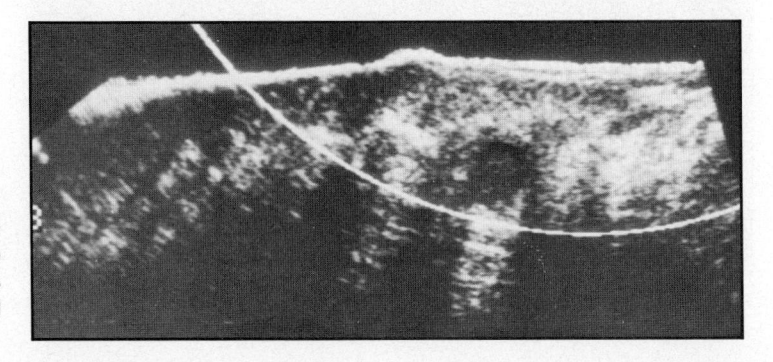

Figure 8-5F. A repeat scan with the mass in the focal zone confirms the presence of the hypoechoic mass and shows through-transmission of sound distally.

Solution:

The mediolateral x-ray mammogram shows vascular calcifications and a bilateral increase in density in both upper hemispheres. However, a bilaterally asymmetric increase in density is present in the left subareolar region (Figure 8-5E). Ultrasonography over the area confirmed the presence of a hypoechoic mass with irregular margins and enhancement of distal echoes (Figure 8-5F). Although distal echo enhancement is more often associated with a cyst than a carcinoma, the presence of echoes in the mass is atypical of a cyst. Moreover, the irregular margin in the ultrasound images suggests the possibility of carcinoma. Biopsy revealed infiltrating carcinoma.

Problem 6:

A 30-year-old woman felt a lump in her left breast. X-ray mammography was negative. An ultrasound examination was performed (Figure 8-6).

quiz cases **167**

Figure 8-6A.

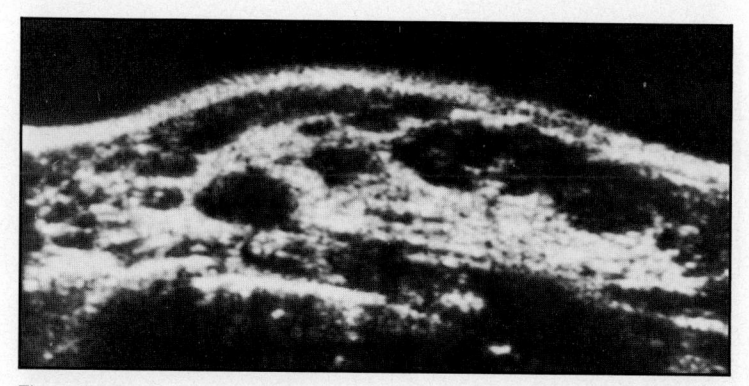

Figure 8-6B.

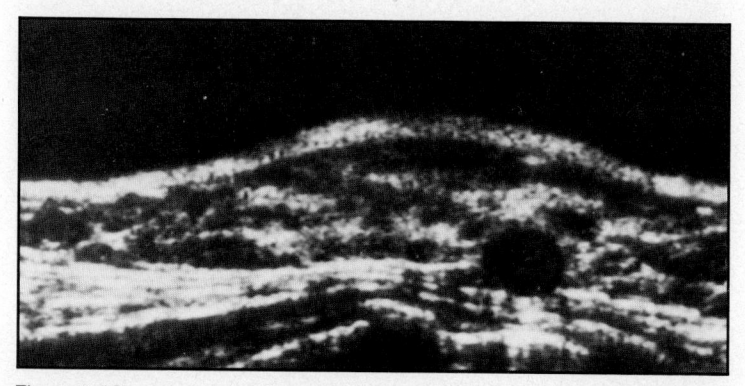

Figure 8-6C.

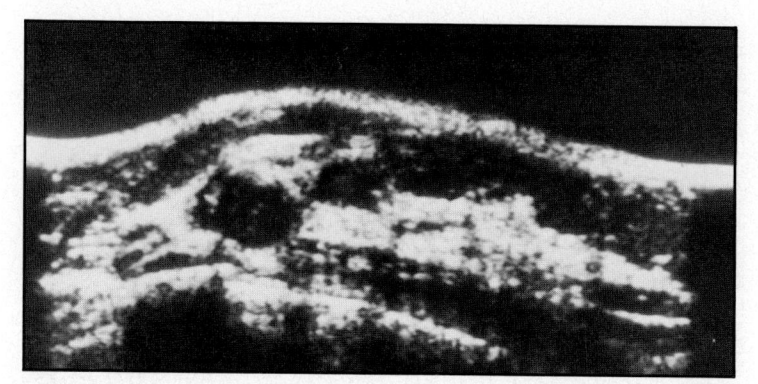

Figure 8-6A,B,C. The automated ultrasound examination includes two transverse sections (A,B) 6mm apart, and one longitudinal section (C) from the same area. (Labsonics)

168 breast ultrasound

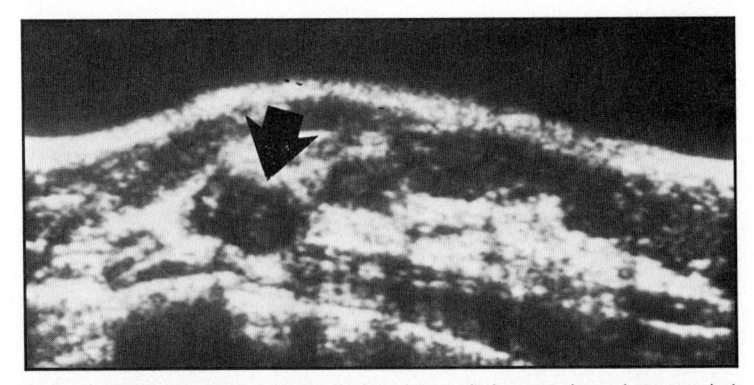

Figure 8-6D. Transverse sections disclose hypoechoic mass (arrow) surrounded by fat lobules.

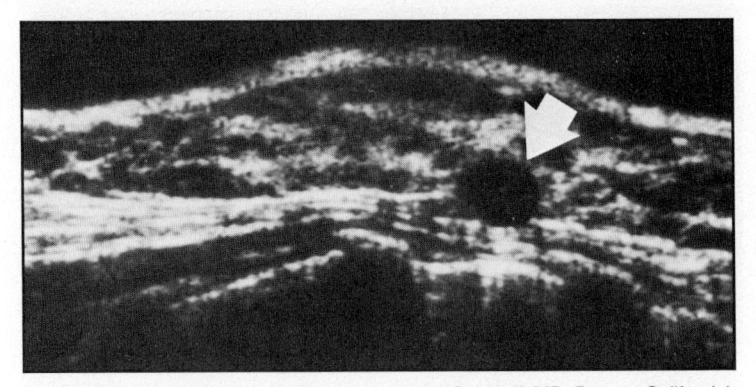

Figure 8-6E. Longitudinal scan. (Courtesy of Joel Sokoloff, MD, Poway, California)

Solution:

A well-circumscribed hypoechoic mass is located anterior to the chest wall. On the transverse images it would have been difficult to differentiate the mass from surrounding fat lobules had the fat lobules not changed shape from one section to the next (Figure 8-6D). The longitudinal scan image confirmed the presence of the hypoechoic mass (Figure 8-6E). Needle aspiration was not attempted because the mass had features of a solid lesion, necessitating biopsy. Excision biopsy revealed fibroadenoma.

Problem 7:

A 79-year-old woman complained of a lump in the upper-outer quadrant of her right breast. X-ray mammography and hand-held ultrasonography were performed (Figure 8-7).

quiz cases   **171**

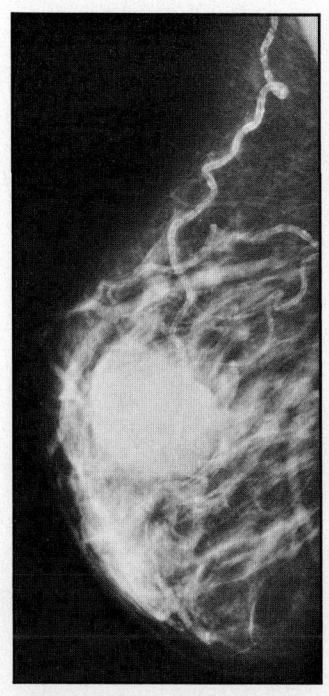

Figure 8-7A. Oblique x-ray mammogram of the right breast.

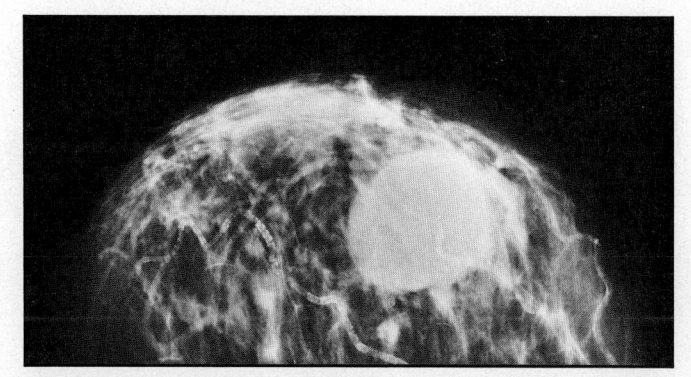

Figure 8-7B. Cephalocaudal x-ray mammogram of the right breast.

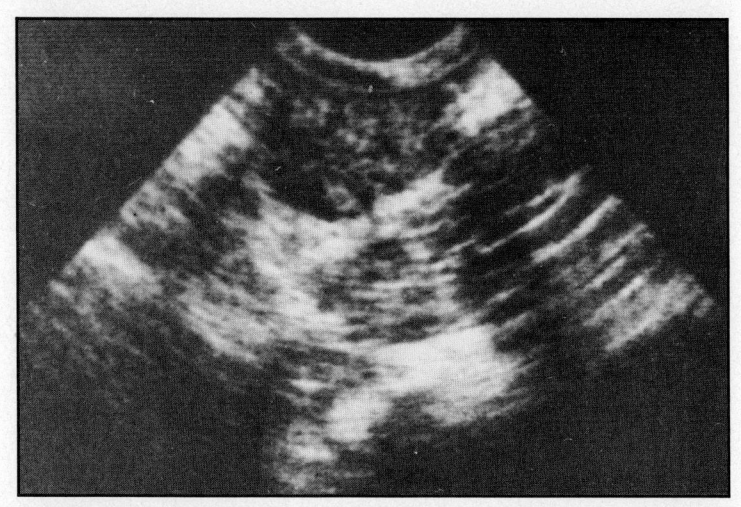

Figure 8-7C. Hand-held ultrasound image.

172 *breast ultrasound*

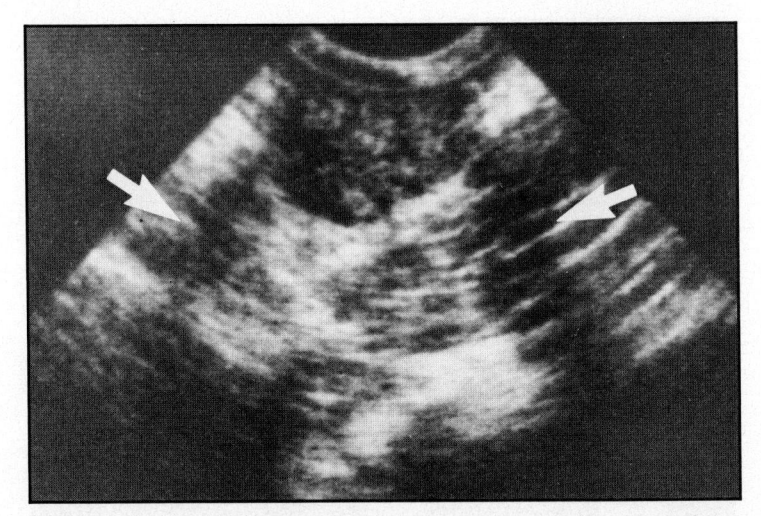

Figure 8-7D. Hand-held ultrasonography over the palpable mass shows homogeneous medium-level echoes and lateral edge refraction (arrows).

Solution:

Although the x-ray mammograms depict a mass with benign features, a well-circumscribed carcinoma must still be considered foremost because of the patient's age. Since the ultrasound examination showed that the mass was solid (Figure 8-7D), aspiration was not performed. Biopsy revealed papillary carcinoma.

Problem 8:

A 43-year-old woman was referred for evaluation of multiple masses in the right breast. Previous aspiration of a similar mass in the same breast yielded clear fluid. X-ray mammography and automated breast ultrasonography were performed (Figure 8-8).

quiz cases 175

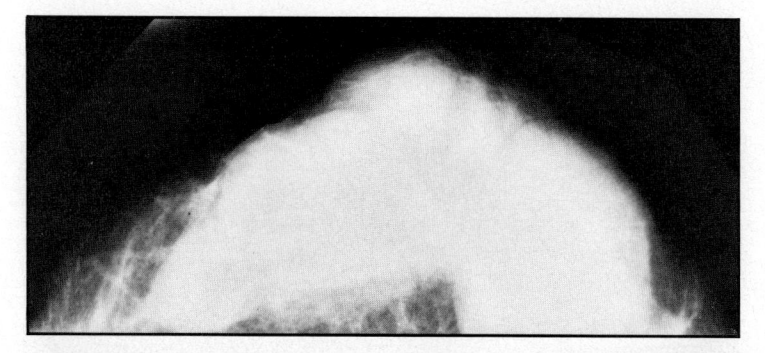

Figure 8-8A. Right cephalo-caudal x-ray mammogram.

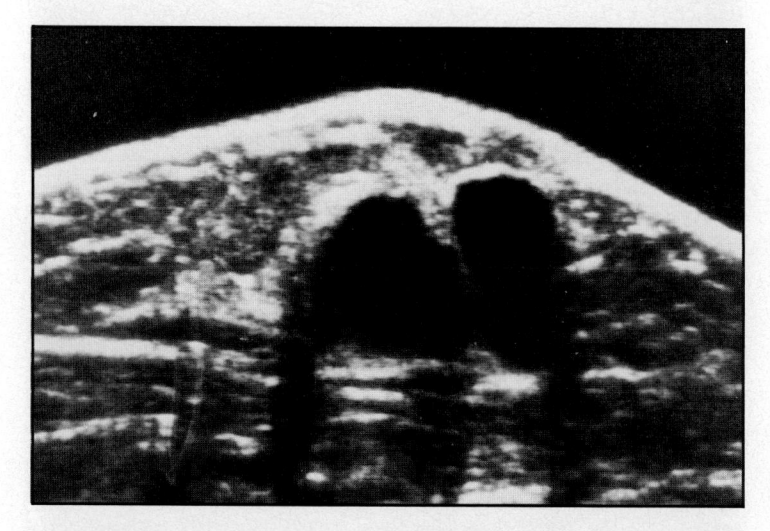

Figure 8-8B. Automated ultrasound section from the upper-inner quadrant of the right breast. (Labsonics)

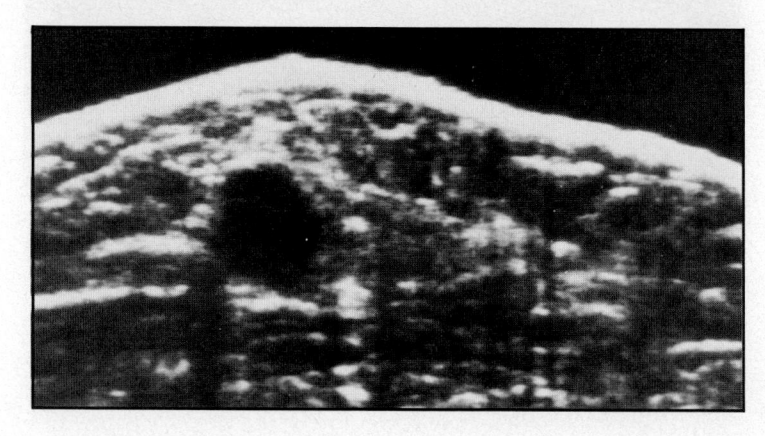

Figure 8-8C. Automated ultrasound section from the upper-inner quadrant of the right breast. (Labsonics)

176 breast ultrasound

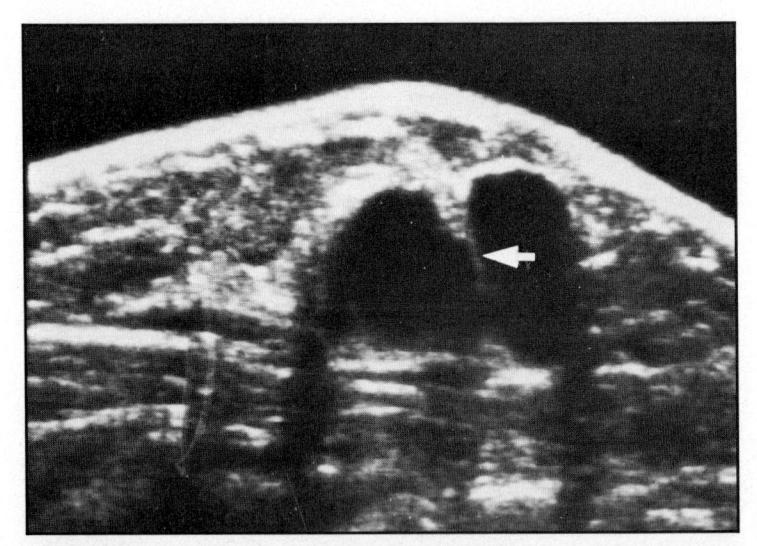

Figure 8-8D. Ultrasound reveals paired cysts separated by a septum (arrow). The cysts are characterized by smooth margins, anechoic interiors, and lateral edge refraction.

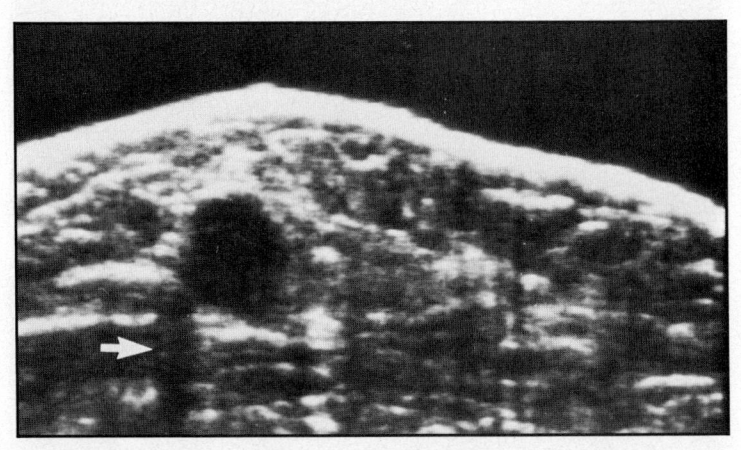

Figure 8-8E. Another ultrasound section discloses an adjacent solid mass. Features are interior echoes, less well-defined margins, and lateral edge refraction (arrow). (Courtesy of Wende Logan, MD, Buffalo, New York)

Solution:

The x-ray mammogram depicts a dense breast with several large masses. Ultrasonography reveals two large anechoic masses in one section (Figure 8-8D). At aspiration, these proved to be communicating cysts. In another section there is a hypoechoic mass that is not as well-circumscribed as the cysts (Figure 8-8E). Because aspiration of the mass yielded no fluid, an excisional biopsy was performed, revealing an infiltrating carcinoma manifesting extensive necrosis.

Problem 9:

A 44-year-old woman with a "cystic" right breast had a left mastectomy for carcinoma three years ago. She is now referred for routine x-ray mammography. X-ray mammographic and breast ultrasound examinations are presented.

quiz cases   179

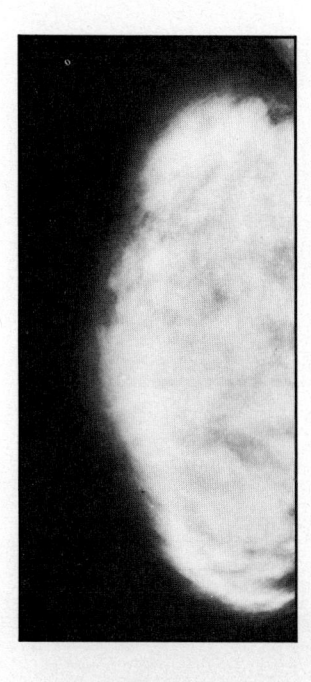

Figure 8-9A. Mediolateral x-ray mammogram of right breast.

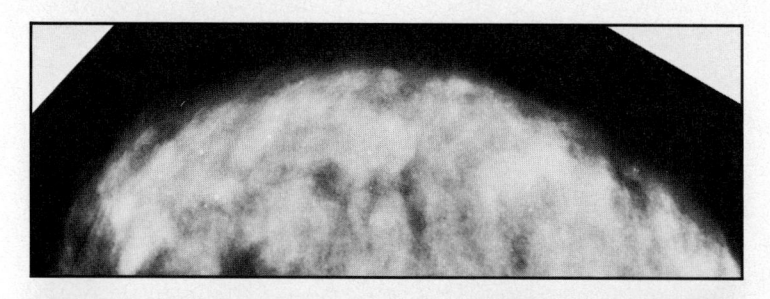

Figure 8-9B. Cephalocaudal x-ray mammogram of right breast.

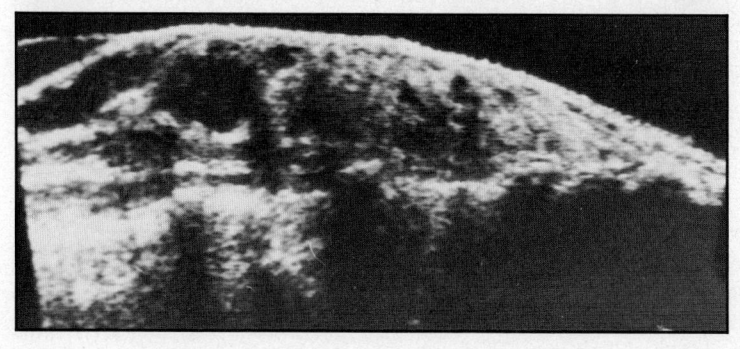

Figure 8-9C. Longitudinal section, automated whole-breast ultrasound, with compression. (Ausonics)

180 breast ultrasound

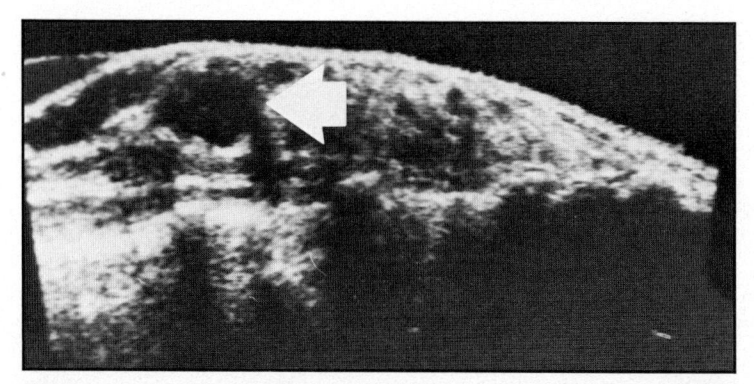

Figure 8-9D. Ultrasound reveals sonolucent mass (arrow) with irregular borders and containing a few low-level echoes. Lateral edge refraction and central through-transmission are present.

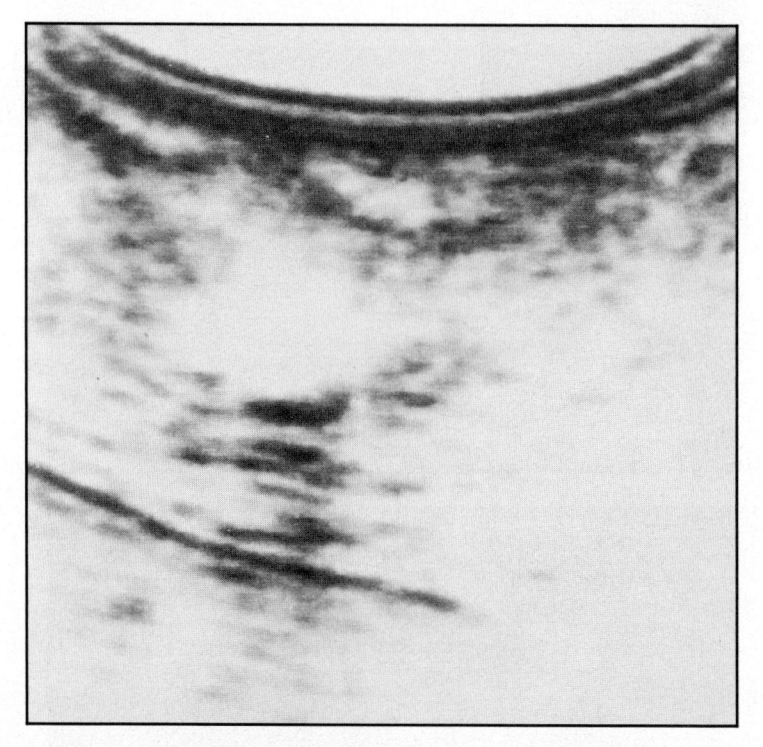

Figure 8-9E. Hand-held real-time ultrasonography performed at time of fine needle aspiration discloses poorly defined boundaries of mass, but does not depict internal echoes.

Solution:

The x-ray mammograms reveal only strikingly dense parenchyma containing scattered microcalcifications. Because the usefulness of the x-ray mammograms was limited by the increased density of the parenchyma, automated whole-breast ultrasonography was performed, disclosing a nonpalpable solid mass (Figure 8-9D). Because there is no reliable ultrasound criterion to distinguish a solid benign mass from a malignant one, fine needle aspiration of the mass was performed under real-time ultrasound guidance (Figure 8-9E), revealing malignant cells. Subsequent excisional biopsy disclosed an intraductal carcinoma that would have gone undetected without ultrasonography.

Problem 10:
A 34-year-old woman felt a lump in the upper-outer quadrant of her right breast. X-ray mammograms and hand-held breast ultrasonograms were performed.

quiz cases 183

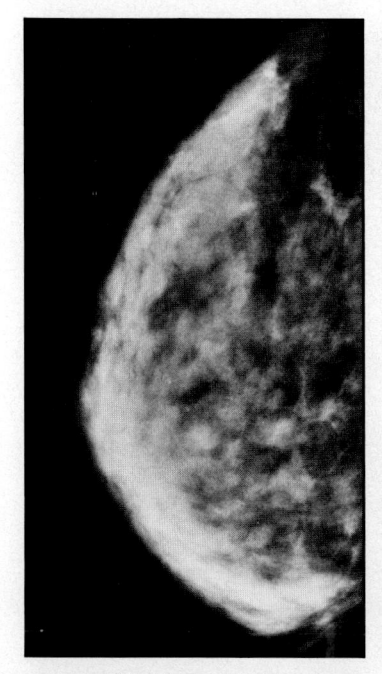

Figure 8-10A. Right mediolateral x-ray mammogram.

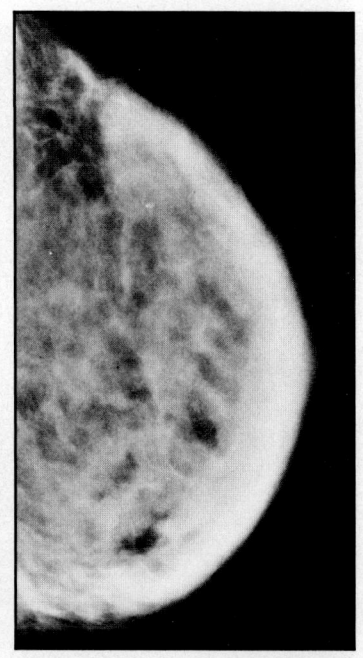

Figure 8-10B. Left mediolateral x-ray mammogram.

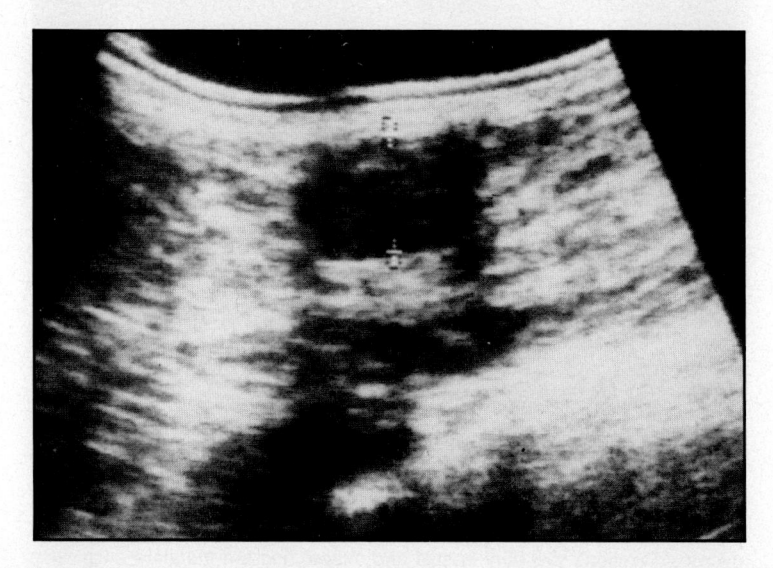

Figure 8-10C. Hand-held real-time examination over the palpable breast mass.

184 breast ultrasound

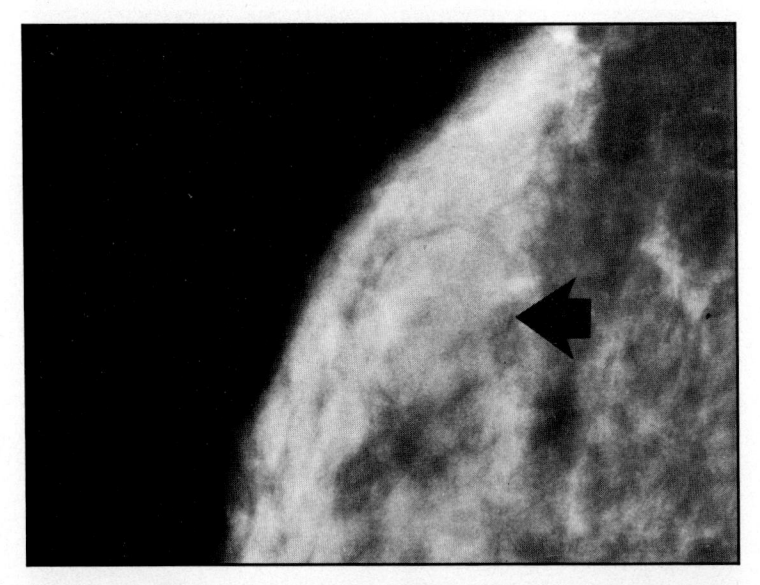

Figure 8-10D. X-ray mammogram of the right breast reveals that the palpable mass is lobulated and surrounded by a thin radiolucent halo.

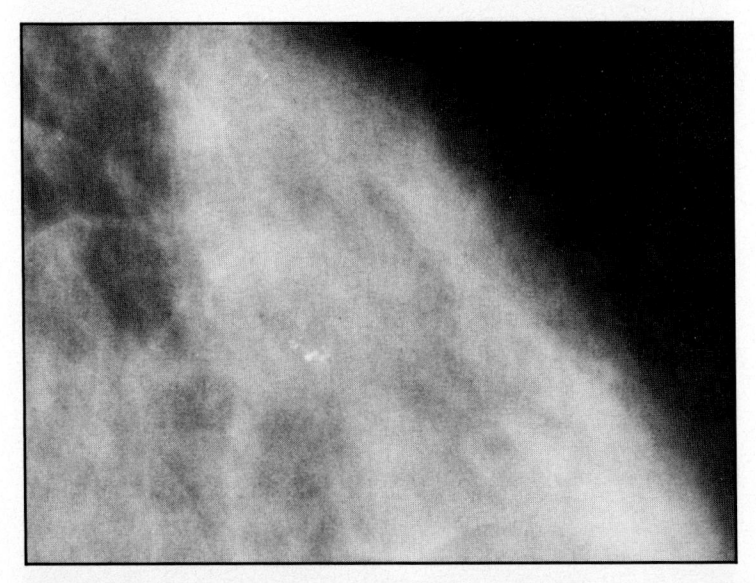

Figure 8-10E. X-ray mammogram of the left breast discloses a cluster of microcalcifications that vary in size and shape, and are therefore suspicious for malignancy.

Solution:

In retrospect, the x-ray mammogram of the right breast depicts a well-circumscribed mass in the upper hemisphere at the site of the palpable abnormality. The surrounding thin radiolucent halo suggests a benign lesion such as a cyst or fibroadenoma (Figure 8-10D). The ultrasound findings of a solid well-circumscribed mass, correlated with the findings on x-ray mammography, is further evidence of a fibroadenoma; this diagnosis was confirmed by biopsy. However, the x-ray mammogram of the left breast discloses a cluster of suspicious calcifications in the upper hemisphere (Figure 8-10E). Biopsy following needle localization revealed a small nonpalpable focus of intraductal carcinoma. This curable cancer would not have been detected if the x-ray mammograms had not been performed.

APPENDIX

Physics and Instrumentation Terms Defined

Absorption
That part of the process of attenuation that cannot be depicted in the image. (Scattering, the other component of attenuation, produces a fine texture). *Absorption* depends on the density, temperature, elasticity, and molecular structure of the attenuating medium. *Classic absorption* is due mainly to heat created by the molecules bumping against each other as they transmit the mechanical wave.

Acoustic Gel
A jelly-like, clear, water-soluble material placed between the breast and the transducer (or water bag) to exclude air from the surface of the transducer. The air is unwanted because it stops the ultrasound transmission and causes black streaks in the image.

AIUM
The American Institute of Ultrasound in Medicine, a professional society. The *100mm AIUM test object* is used for quality control.

A-Line
The rectified signal of one pulse of ultrasound returning to the transducer from reflectors and scatterers in the breast. These echoes are usually amplified and compensated for attenuation before being displayed as an A-line. A-lines (or A-mode transmission) were once used for diagnosis, especially to detect a lateral shift of the midline structures of the brain. Now they mainly help adjust the time gain compensation controls and verify that the interiors of cysts are echo-free.

Amplitude
The height of the A-line signal, or the amount of voltage generated in the transducer when the returning echoes strike the piezoelectric wafer.

Anechoic
Without echoes, as in a fluid filled cyst. Because an anechoic region may absorb ultrasound but does not scatter ultrasound, it attenuates less than other regions.

Angle of Incidence

The angle at which the ultrasound beam strikes a tissue interface. The amount of reflection is decreased as the angle of incidence shifts from 90°.

Attenuation

The decrease in the amplitude and intensity of the beam due to absorption and scattering. Attenuation increases with frequency, so that a 3.5MHz beam has one-half the dB attenuation of a 7MHz beam. Attenuation is measured in decibels (dB).

Axial Resolution

The ability to resolve two interfaces that are perpendicular to the direction of the beam. Axial resolution depends on transducer frequency, damping of the pulse as it leaves the transducer, matching layer between the piezoelectric wafer and breast, frequency bandwidth of the amplifiers, output power, and amount of amplification.

Azimuthal Resolution (Lateral Resolution)

The ability to resolve two objects in the same plane beneath the transducer when the plane is parallel to the face of the transducer. Azimuthal resolution is poorer than axial resolution. It is mainly controlled by the transducer focal lens (or phasing of array transducers) and is useful only to a depth 4cm to 5cm for transducers used in breast imaging.

Beam

The pulsed ultrasonic wave, consisting of three to four cycles of ultrasound.

Beam Width

A synonym for the lateral resolution of round-faced transducers. Beam width is also loosely used to refer to the cross-sectional area of the ultrasound pulse as it moves away from the transducer.

B-Mode

Brightness mode, a conventional static (as opposed to

real-time) image. The technologist moves a transducer across the patient to form a single frame. The returning amplitudes are assigned to gray levels in the image.

Calipers

The electronic calipers that are moved with a joy stick or by depression of arrows on the keyboard to measure a distance in the displayed image. Their accuracy depends on the velocity of sound in the breast and on the calibration of the motor that moves the transducer (or on the phasing of an array of transducers).

Compound Image

This occurs in the following manner: If the digital memory that contains the image is not erased between frames or is not replaced by a new frame filling the memory location, but instead each memory element compares the new echo amplitude to the previous one already stored in that location and retains the larger of the two values, the resulting image is called a compound image. Compound imaging is particularly useful when more than one transducer forms the image.

Contrast

This refers to the difference in the amount of amplitude between the gray levels in an image. If the image is composed only of black and white, its contrast is maximum; an image composed of white and light gray has poor contrast. The contrast can be changed by changing the gray scale map used to represent the ultrasound amplitudes.

Critical Angle

A refractive phenomenon occurs when the ultrasound beam refracts off a surface that is curved beyond its critical angle and therefore does not penetrate the surface. Should the upper surface of the curve have a lower velocity of sound than the lower surface, the refraction will be complete.

Decibel

A unit of measurement of the ratio of two wave amplitudes. This is the unit used in the calibration of the intensity, amplitude, or power of an initial ultrasound wave relative to its attenuated value. For voltages, attenuation is measured in decibels (dB) by the formula $20 \log_{10}(A_2/A_1)$, where A_1 is the incident voltage and A_2 is the received voltage.

Diffraction
This refers to to the cause of scattering, a component of attenuation. The beam is not only diffracted by passing through a finite aperture (the transducer), but each tissue cell along its path diffracts the beam if the cell diameter is smaller than two or three wavelengths.

Digital
The signal returns to the transducer as a continuous voltage; however, a computer memory requires discrete values. These discrete values are referred to as digital, and are derived from the continuous changes in voltage by means of the thresholding and comparison of steps, a process called *digitization*.

Doppler
This refers to the velocity of tissue, but actually represents the velocity of the circulating blood within it. The ultrasound changes frequency when reflected from moving tissue. The amount that the tissue moves can be calculated from this frequency change by the doppler instrument.

Dynamic Range
The lowest and highest voltages that can be received by the ultrasound equipment. This determines the penetration of the ultrasound. Some units change their gray scale maps by reducing the dynamic range. This is accomplished by assigning large echoes to a single gray level value, and assigning low level echoes to a broader range of gray levels. While the contrast is increased for small voltage echoes, this is not really a reduction in dynamic range, since the large echoes still appear in the image.

Elasticity
The stiffness or lack of compliance of tissue. This

determines the velocity at which sound travels through it. The stiffer or more elastic the tissue, the greater the velocity. Elasticity affects the attenuation and reflection of sound in tissue.

Far Field

The region beyond the focal zone where the beam loses intensity and spreads. The amount of spreading is least for unfocused high frequency transducers. High frequency transducers are usually sharply focused, causing the far field to diverge and weaken abruptly.

Filtering

The process of removing some frequencies from the received voltage wave form. Noise is often of high or low frequency and may be removed by filtering those frequencies from the received signal to improve the image. Frequencies that are not part of the bandwidth, having been introduced by the equipment, may also be filtered.

Focal Zone

The area where the beam is narrowest, producing the best lateral resolution, thinnest slice, and most intense amplitude. In focused transducers, the closer the focus is to the transducer, the shorter the focal zone. Small cysts and solid lesions can be obscured or misdiagnosed if they are not imaged in the focal zone.

Frame Rate

The speed at which the image changes in a real-time unit. Real-time breast scanning helps the mammographer to visualize a three-dimensional volume. If the frame rate is below 20 frames/sec, the image will flicker between frames. However, 30 frames/second are not needed to achieve a smooth transition from frame to frame. Indeed, by reducing the frame rate and penetration depth, more lines per frame can be processed, resulting in a superior image.

Frequency

The number of cycles per second in the ultrasound wave. The cycle is formed from each rarefaction and amplification of the particles transmitting the wave. The length of the cycle is called a wave length. The frequency is proportional to the wave length, which is computed from the velocity of the wave in a particular tissue. The unit of measurement of frequency is the Hertz (Hz). Thus, 1MHz (megaHertz) is 1 million cycles/sec.

Frequency Bandwidth

A mixture of frequencies that emerge from the transducer. Since this mixture is usually nearly Gaussian or bell-shaped, it is the peak frequency that is marked on the transducer. The range of frequencies on both sides of the peak value is the frequency bandwidth. Due to the increased attenuation of higher frequencies in tissue, the peak frequency decreases in the frequency bandwidth as the beam moves farther from the transducer and deeper into tissue (but not in water). Since the high frequency components help to image the finer structures, the attenuation of the high frequencies causes diminished resolution with increasing penetration of the breast.

Gain

The amplification applied to the received voltage. Since amplification is also applied to noise, too much gain can create artifacts in anechoic regions by filling them with amplified noise.

Gray Scale (Gray Map)

Each received level of voltage is assigned to a unique gray level. The distribution of voltage levels where these thresholds occur is called a gray scale or gray map. This threshold table more than any other factor affects the presentation of texture.

Impedance (Acoustic)

The property of tissue, dependent on its density and stiffness, that controls the reflection of the ultrasound wave between tissue structures. A large difference in the impedance of two adjacent structures will cause a large reflection. Air stops ultrasound dramatically because of the large difference between its impedance and that of the adjacent tissue.

Intensity (sonic intensity or power)
The amount of power applied to a transducer to generate an incident ultrasound wave.

Lateral Resolution
See Azimuthal Resolution.

Linear Array
An array of many small transducers arranged in a line. Each transducer is pulsed with the adjacent ones so that 10 to 30 transducers may be fired at once to produce one "beam" of ultrasound. These individual wavelets of sound interact like the wave from a single large transducer. They are focused in the slice thickness direction with an external ultrasound lens placed on each wafer.

Lobes
Side lobes are produced by all transducers and are the result of wavelet interactions. They are low in amplitude and do not affect the image unless very low level echoes are amplified. Grating lobes occur with arrays of transducers, but will not affect the image so long as the separation between the centers of separate transducers is less than a wavelength.

Log Amp (Logarithmic Amplifier)
Small echoes are amplified more than large ones.

Moire Pattern
A circular wave-like pattern in the digital image due to an under-sampling of the data. The pattern will be less obvious if additional scan lines are formed by interpolating them between the original scan lines.

Piezoelectric
The physical property of generating a voltage when struck with a mechanical wave. The ceramic wafers in most transducers consists of lead zirconate titanate (PZT), a

man-made material that is made piezoelectric by heating and then cooling it under a uniform voltage.

Phased Array
A linear array in which the adjacent transducers are not fired together, but with a delay so that the wavelets constructively interfere at a known focal distance. Alternatively, received waves from a specified distance can be delayed to simulate a focused returning wave.

Posterior Enhancement versus Posterior Shadowing
If the area behind or posterior to a lesion is *enhanced*, the ultrasound beam was not attenuated as much as the time gain compensation amplified it. Thus the lesion is either cystic or composed of a tissue less dense and elastic than the surrounding breast tissue. If the area posterior to the lesion exhibits *shadowing*, increased attenuation occurred in the lesion, and it must be stiffer and denser than the surrounding breast tissue.

Postprocessing
When gray levels are reassigned from those in the digital memory at the time of the image display. If more than 15 gray levels were assigned at the time of digitization, reassigning them according to some other gray level map may enhance the image.

Power
See Intensity.

Preprocessing
Gray level assignments to specific voltage levels before digitization. If a compound image is formed rather than a survey image, this decision is also considered a preprocessing one.

Range
The depth of penetration of the ultrasound wave. Some ultrasound units ignore signals reflected from nondiagnostic ranges. Since range is limited in breast imaging, the real-time unit's tradeoff between range, frames/

sec, and number of lines/frame allows breast imaging equipment to process more lines per frame.

Real Time
The automatic movement of the transducer or pulses of ultrasound to form an image. Real-time imaging allows the visualization of moving tissue in the body or, in the case of the breast, allows a three-dimensional visualization by rapidly displaying successive slices.

Reflection
The return of part of the ultrasound beam from a broad smooth surface. The surface represents an impedance mismatch between two tissues. Unlike *optical* reflection, *acoustic* reflection depends on both the velocity and density of the two media. When more of the wave is reflected, less is transmitted; thus less of the ultrasound beam is available to image deeper structures.

Refraction
The beam bending between two tissues with different velocities, when the interface between the two tissues is not perpendicular to the beam's incident direction of travel. See critical angle.

Reverberbations
Artifactual echoes resulting from the unit "painting in" echoes that have re-reflected off hard surfaces such as the transducer, water bath membrane, or skin.

Scan Converter
The computer memory that contains the digitized wave forms assembled into an array of numbers representing the different gray levels. The locations of the numbers in the memory represent the locations of the gray levels in the image.

Scattering
The component of attenuation that is responsible for texture in the ultrasound image. Like absorption, scattering is affected by frequency, density, and elasticity, but it is also affected by tissue cell diameter and the spacings

between the cells, which act as diffraction gratings upon the ultrasound waves.

Sector Scan (Sector Image)
An image shaped like a wedge of pie. The scan is formed by a real-time transducer wobbling back and forth to form an image. Phased arrays can also be guided to form sector images.

Signal Processing
The operations applied to the received voltage wave forms before they are stored in the digital scan convertor. These operations may consist of amplification, time gain compensation (TGC), demodulation (or simple rectification and/or envelope detection), filtering, sampling, digitizing, peak detection, thresholding, and gray level assignment.

Slice Thickness
The elevation resolution of each image. Unlike computerized tomography, where each image section represents a uniform thickness of the patient's body, ultrasound slice thickness varies with beam resolution. Thus for round transducers it follows the lateral resolution measurements. For phased or linear arrays, since each element is focused with a fixed focus external lens, the slice thickness varies with the characteristics of this lens. In the far field, small lesions may not be imaged because of the partial volume effect.

Slope
The amount of TGC applied with increasing depth. Higher frequency transducers attenuate at a faster rate and require a steeper TGC slope.

Speckle
The fine grain shimmering texture resulting from the effects of diffraction in an ultrasound image.

Specular Surface
A surface that is large and smooth. In ultrasound, this is represented by any interface between two tissues that

is more than ten wavelengths in diameter, so that reflection relationships rather than scattering relationships control the behavior of the ultrasound wave.

Static
An image that does not change over time. A B-mode image is a static image.

Survey
The type of image resulting from scanning with one transducer while the digital scan converter memory continually replaces old memory values with the new values from the current scan. See Compound.

TGC
Time gain compensation. Since attenuation increases with depth, echoes returning from deep within the breast need increased amplification, which is assigned by the TGC.

Thread Target (Thread Test Object)
Used for quality control to assess lateral and axial resolution. By scanning across evenly spaced threads, the changes in beam diameter with depth can be imaged for lateral resolution calibration. Similarly, if the parallel threads are arranged so that their spacing becomes progressively narrower, axial resolution can be measured.

Transducer
A device that acts to send and receive the ultrasound wave. It consists primarily of a piezoelectric wafer and focusing material.

Velocity
The speed of ultrasonic propagation in tissue. Most North American ultrasound units assume that this is 1540m/sec.

Wave Length
The length of the cycle formed from each rarefaction and amplification of the particles transmitting the sound wave.

INDEX

Abduction 48, 49
Abnormality 100
 Focal 113
 Palpable 4, 97, 118
 Pathologic vii
 Sonographic 4
 X-ray 131
Abscess 83, 98, 106
Absorption 15, 25, 26, 95, 113, 189, 190, 197
 Ultrasound 25
Acini 90, 91
Acuson phased array 47
Adenosis
 Sclerosing 135, 136
A-line 28, 86, 189
Aluminum plate 17
American Institute of Ultrasound Medicine (AIUM) 189
A-mode vii, 3, 189
Amplification 27, 38, 44, 189, 190, 193-196, 198, 199
 Electrical 17
 Linear 40
Amplitude 19, 24, 29, 40, 44, 53, 67, 75, 189-194
Ampulla 67
Angiosarcoma 125, 126
Annular array transducer 8
Areola 63, 66-68, 86, 98, 134
Arm 55, 118
 Ipsilateral 48, 49
 Scanning 57
Armamentarium
 Radiologic viii
Array 47, 195
 Annular transducer 8
 Electrically-driven 41
 Element 47
 Linear 47, 195, 196, 198
 Phased 46, 47, 196, 198
  Acuson 47
 Transducer 190
 Ultrasound 191
 Unit 46
Artifact 17, 27, 29, 30, 43, 44, 46, 137, 141, 194, 197
 Mechanical real-time 43
 Phased array 46
 Reverberation 16, 42
Aspiration 3, 50, 51, 87, 90, 120
 Biopsy 6, 49, 131
 Cyst 90
 Needle 3, 5, 6, 49, 86, 131
 Ultrasound-guided 5, 6
Attenuation 24-27, 29, 37, 59, 65, 67, 75, 92, 94, 98, 99, 105, 111, 113, 114, 126, 131, 133, 137, 189, 190, 192-194, 196-199

Ausonics (unit) 47, 53-55, 57, 59, 66, 68, 69, 71, 73, 74, 78, 86, 88, 103-105, 114, 115, 132, 141
Axilla 57
Axillary tail 48, 49
Backscatter 7
Baseline
 Ultrasonic 48
Baum 3
Beam 19, 23, 24, 33, 43, 44, 59, 70, 133, 140, 141, 190, 192-195, 197-199
 Filtration 18
 On-axis 44
 Sound 57, 99
 Transducer 137
 Ultrasound 19, 33, 65, 67, 70, 75, 111, 133, 190, 191, 196, 197
Benign disorder 81-106
Biopsy 3, 5, 6, 50, 90, 94, 99-102, 112, 114, 118, 131, 133, 136
 Aspiration 6, 49, 131
 Breast viii, 132
 Needle 6, 49, 131
 Ultrasound-guided 5
B-mode 3, 23, 42, 56, 57, 190, 199
Brain 25
Breast vii-ix, 3-8, 16-19, 21-27, 29, 32, 33, 37, 42-44, 46-49, 51-53, 55, 57, 58, 61-79, 83-86, 90, 93, 94, 96-101, 103-105, 109, 111-115, 137, 139, 141, 189-191, 193, 194, 197, 199
Atrophic 95
Augmentation
 Mammoplasty 83, 104
 Prostheses 5
Biopsy viii, 132
Cancer 4, 5, 109, 131
Carcinoma 109, 113, 115, 117
Cyst 24
Dedicated unit 37
 Automated 7
Dense 5, 7, 8, 109, 113, 137
 Nodular fibrocystic 5
Disease vii, viii
Dysplastic 27
Examination 15, 49
Fatty 4, 70, 72, 95, 109, 123, 133, 134
Fibrocystic 5, 27
Glandular 27
Imaging viii, x, 16, 24, 38, 42, 44, 46, 54, 55, 190, 196, 197
 Real-time 151

Implant 103
Lactating 67, 99
Lesion 83
Lump 109
Lumpy 86
Male 137, 140, 141
Malignancy 109
Mass vii, 3, 70, 75, 113, 136
 Palpable ix
 Solid 3
Metastases 125
Multinodular 90
Parenchyma ix, 111
Penetration 16
Pregnant 78
RMI phantom 58
Tissue vii, viii, 8, 15, 16, 24, 25, 37, 38, 59, 95, 104, 111, 117, 135, 137, 196
Calcification 17, 90, 97
Caliper 50, 191
 Electronic 49, 59, 191
Cancer viii, 8, 17, 90, 109, 133, 134
 Breast 4, 5, 109, 131
 Metastatic 125
 Noncalcified 5
 Nonpalpable 4
 Subareolar 66
Capsule 29, 30, 86, 87, 90, 92, 93, 95, 97, 98, 106
 Cyst 29, 33
Carcinoma 7, 8, 109-111, 113, 115-118, 120, 136
 Colloid 116, 120, 123
 Ductal 118
  Infiltrating 109-114, 117, 120
 Infiltrating 111
  Ductal 109-114, 117, 120
  Lobular 119
 Lobular 117
  Infiltrating 119
 Medullary 116, 117, 119, 120
 Mucinous 120
 Papillary 116, 120-122
Cell 26, 110, 122, 198
 Epithelial 95, 120
 Tumor 111
 Memory 41
 Tissue 192, 197
Ceramic
 Lead zirconate titanate (PZT) 18
 Wafer 195
Chemotherapy 124
Chest 21, 22, 27, 28, 67, 87, 140, 141
Cleft 90-92
Cole-Beuglet 113
Collagen 8

Collagenosis 75
Compression 37, 51, 53, 55, 57, 65-67, 69-71, 73, 75, 78, 84, 88, 89, 96, 102, 103, 137-139
Computer 18, 22, 37, 40, 41, 57, 192, 197
Computerized tomography 198
Contrast 40, 41
Converter
 Digital scan 18, 26
Cooper's ligaments 63, 65, 67, 70, 71, 111, 133, 135
Cyst viii, 3-5, 26-31, 33, 38, 44, 46, 50, 57, 83-87, 89, 90, 92, 95, 97-99, 101, 120, 122, 137, 189, 193
 Aspiration 90
 Breast 26
 Fluid 3, 29
 Nonpalpable 6, 84, 87, 90
 Palpable 90
 Sebaceous 83, 99, 101
 Septated 88
 Subareolar 86
Cystic disease 5, 90
Cystosarcoma 95
 Phylloides 83, 92
Defect
 Filling 95, 97
Deland 3
Demodulation 198
Desmoplasia 113
Diagnosis 3, 7, 25, 37-39, 46-48, 53, 83, 86, 106, 111, 118, 131, 135, 189, 193, 196
Digital memory 196
Digital scan converter (DSC) 18, 26, 40
 Memory storage table 41, 44
 Storage algorithm 46
Digitization 40, 41, 192, 196, 198
Dilatation 67, 68, 83
Discharge 95, 97
Disease
 Benign vii
 Breast vii, viii
 Cystic 5, 90
 Fibrocystic 86
 Malignant vii
Disfiguration 133
Display mode 41
Distribution
 Bell-shaped 17, 194
 Gaussian 17, 194
Doppler 8, 192
Duct 38, 63, 67, 75, 77, 78, 85,

90, 91, 95, 97, 99, 109-111, 116, 118, 120, 133, 135
Dilated 97
Lactiferous 63, 67
Subareolar 66, 68
Terminal 83
Ductogram 97
Dynamic range 40, 192
Dysplasia 77
Echo 8, 15, 16, 18, 26-31, 38-43, 55, 66, 67, 69, 70, 72, 73, 75, 78, 83, 84, 86, 87, 89, 92-100, 103, 104, 109, 111-113, 117-120, 123-126, 132, 137, 189, 191, 192, 195, 197, 199
Artifactual 23, 197
Background patterns viii
Distal 85-87, 93, 95, 97, 113, 114, 117, 119, 126
Parenchymal 84, 109, 115
Pulse scanner 8
Skin 73
Tissue 18
Ultrasound 44
Echogenicity 70, 109
Echography 66
Breast 8
Egan 113
Electricity 18
Energy
  Mechanical 17
  Reflection 15
  Source 15
  Transmission 15
  Wave 15
Eosin 110, 116
Epithelium 90, 92, 95, 117
Examination 5, 6, 37, 53, 55, 57, 86, 113, 117, 131, 135
Ausonics 68
  Bilateral 55
Automated 141
Bilateral 55, 57
Breast 15, 49, 69, 131, 140
Cytological 50
Dedicated 68
False-negative 133
False-positive 133
Hand-held 21, 68, 69, 85, 93, 94, 98, 100, 118, 137, 141
Mammographic 6, 104
Real-time 21, 57, 68, 85, 87, 88, 93, 97, 98, 100, 118, 137, 141
Sonographic 99
Ultrasound 6, 37, 70, 104, 106, 131, 132
Water-path 137
X-ray 90, 104
Exposure 18
False-negative
  Examination 133
  Ultrasound 134
False-positive
  Examination 133
  Sonography 135

Fascia 63, 75, 125
  Superficial 63
Fat 4, 25, 27, 29, 40, 48, 63, 65, 70, 72, 75, 76, 95, 98, 109, 111, 113, 123, 131, 133-135, 137
  Lobule 63, 67, 70, 75
  Retromammary (RMF) 75, 78, 96
  Subcutaneous 28, 29, 65, 67, 70, 78, 111, 113, 115
  Globule 69
Fiber 70, 76, 117
Fibroadenoma 27, 39, 47, 83, 89-94, 96, 102, 131
Fibrocystic
  Breast 5
  Disease 86
Fibrosis 75, 77, 113
Filling defect 95, 97
Film 18, 37
Film-screen 4, 17, 118
Mammography 17, 134
Filtration 38, 40
  Beam 18
Focal distance 19, 33, 196
Focal lens 19, 190
Focal point 19
Focal range 46
Focal spot 16
  X-ray tube 16
Focal zone 19-21, 25, 42, 43, 46, 55, 57, 60, 141, 193
Focusing 48, 52, 53, 57, 75, 193, 195, 198, 199
Frame 42, 44
  Jump 44
  Rate 42, 44, 193
Frequency viii, 5, 6, 8, 15, 16, 18, 19, 24-27, 38, 40, 190, 192-194, 197
  Ultrasound 25
Friction 25
Galactocele 83, 99, 100
Gel 43
  Acoustic 47, 48, 189
  Water-soluble 17
  Silicone 103, 104
Gland 25, 29, 70, 72, 75, 135, 137
Globule
  Subcutaneous fat 69
Grant 126
Gray level 40, 41, 53, 55, 191, 192, 194, 196-198
Guidelines
  Biostatic viii
Haagenson 117
Hematoma 83, 99, 102
Hematoxylin 110, 116
Hemorrhage
  Traumatic 131
Howry 3
Hyalinization 90, 92

Imaging 15, 16, 18, 19, 21-24, 26, 32, 37, 40-44, 46, 47, 49-51, 53, 55, 57, 59, 60, 65, 111, 112, 133, 135, 137, 141, 189, 191-199
  Automated ix, 59
  Breast x, 24, 28, 37, 38, 42, 44, 46, 51, 54, 55, 133, 190, 196, 197
  Compound 196
  Detector 17
  Hand-held 49
  Membrane 43
  Memory 18
  Multiple sequential 6
  Real-time 49, 51, 59, 191, 197
  Sonographic 113, 117
  Sonomammographic 66
  Survey 196
  Ultrasound vii-ix, 9, 10, 15, 16, 18, 25, 28, 29, 37, 40, 49, 63, 75, 95, 113, 197, 198
  X-ray 16
  Mammographic 18
Impedance 33, 65, 67, 78, 133, 194, 195, 197
Ultrasound 29
Implant 103, 104, 106
Incision 99
Infiltrating carcinoma 111
  Ductal 109-114, 117, 120
  Lobular 119
Infiltration 109-111
Instrumentation vii, ix, 7, 15, 35-61, 131, 141
  Automated 32, 51-59
    Water-path 6
  Breast imaging x
  Hand-held 32, 42
  Labsonics 59
  Real-time 42, 59
  Ultrasound ix
Investigator 4
Involution 90, 92
Jellins 3
Kaiser 3
Kelly-Fry 3
Kidney 25
Kobayashi 3, 113, 120
Kossoff 3
Kratchowil 3
Labsonics (unit) 56, 59, 77, 87, 112, 141
Lactate 67, 99
Lead zirconate titanate (PZT) 18, 195
Lens 22, 23, 33, 198
  Acoustic 19
  Focal 19
  Focusing 19, 46
  Ultrasound 195
Lesion 6, 8, 19, 26, 32, 33, 38, 40, 41, 43, 44, 49-51, 53, 111, 117, 193, 196, 198
  Anechoic 43, 44, 46

Benign 83, 120
  Breast 83
  Cystic 48, 196
  Malignant 26, 83, 107-127
  Mass 83
  Nonpalpable 5, 6, 48, 49
  Palpable 51, 83
  Solid viii, 4, 44, 48, 83, 120
Ligaments
  Cooper's 63, 65, 67, 70, 71, 111, 133, 135
Light photon 17
Lipoma 83, 95, 97, 98
Liver 25
Lobe
  Grating 46, 47, 195
  Side 44, 195
Lobule 63, 78, 92, 98, 117, 123, 126, 134
  Fat 63, 67, 70, 75, 135
  Mammary 63
  Parechymal 63
Log-amplification 38, 40, 44, 195
Logan, Wende W. 77
Lump 84, 93, 100, 101, 105, 109, 112, 123
  Palpable 48
Lumpectomy 131, 132
Lymphoma
  Non-Hodgkins 124
Malignancy 4, 26, 83, 109, 111, 113, 125, 131, 133, 135, 136
Mammograhy 3-6, 17, 72-74, 76, 77, 84-86, 88, 94, 95, 97, 100, 101, 103, 105, 114, 115, 118, 123, 125, 136, 141, 193
  Film-screen 17, 134
  Ultrasound vii, 4, 16, 75, 137
  Automated 7
  X-ray vii-ix, 4-8, 15-18, 37, 63, 70, 71, 75, 90, 106, 109, 111, 113, 115, 117, 120, 121, 133, 135, 141
Mammoplasty 106
  Breast augmentation 83, 104
Mass 3, 20-22, 27-29, 32, 39, 41, 43, 48, 51, 66, 70, 83-85, 88, 90, 93-101, 109, 112, 114, 115, 117-119, 121-123, 125, 126, 131, 134-137, 141
  Benign 3
  Breast vii, 3, 70, 75, 113, 136
  Palpable ix
  Solid 3
  Carcinoma 109, 113
  Cystic 4, 90, 141
  Fibroepithelial 90
  Fixation 6
  Hypoechoic 112, 114, 115, 136
  Lesion 83
  Lobulated 123
  Malignant 3

index

Mammographic 6
Noncalcified 3
Nonpalpable 3, 5
Palpable 3, 5, 6, 93, 94, 96, 121
  Multiple 7, 88
  Solid viii, 3, 4, 28, 29, 39, 47, 90, 96, 122, 131, 137, 141
    Benign viii, 3, 4, 89, 109, 116, 118
    Malignant viii, 3, 4
  Sonolucent 87
  Subareolar 86, 98
Melanoma 118
Menopause 90, 95
Metastasis 83, 92, 125
Microcalcification 4, 23, 90, 109, 111, 117, 120, 133
Micrometer
  Mechanical 57
Microprocessor 8
Mirror, acoustic 23
Moire wave 41, 195
Morbidity 133
Mucin 8, 120
Mucopolysaccharide 8
Muscle 75
  Pectoralis 63, 65, 67, 69, 102
  Major 75
Near field 15
Necrosis 131
Needle 50, 51
  Aspiration 6, 49, 86, 131
  Biopsy 6, 49, 131
  Prebiopsy
    Localization 5
Nipple 48, 53, 55, 63, 66-68, 74, 95, 97, 114, 115, 135
Nodular fibrocystic breast 5
Nodule 124
Offset 21, 42, 43
  Fluid 42, 43
  Oil 23
  Substance 22, 23
  Water 23, 32, 33, 43, 46, 47
  Water bag 21
Oil 16, 17, 23, 48
Optics 33
Palpation ix, 3, 4, 48, 49, 141
Papilloma 83, 95, 97, 120
Parenchyma 7, 25, 26, 29, 63, 65, 67, 70, 72-76, 78, 84, 93, 95, 99, 109, 111-113, 115, 117, 121, 135
  Breast ix, 111
Parenchymal tissue 7, 111, 133
Penetration 53, 65, 70, 75, 113, 133, 135, 137-139, 191-194, 196
  Breast 16, 27, 75
  Tissue 16, 135
Phantom 59
  RMI breast 58
  Ultrasonic breast 59
Phase 40, 46

Philips (unit) 38, 47
Phosphor 17
Photon 17
Phylloides cystosarcoma 83, 92
Picker microview 47
Piezoelectric 195, 196
  Wafer 18, 24, 33, 189, 190, 199
Pitfall ix, 75, 129-142
Polyethylene 57
Polyvinyl 8
Polyvinylidene fluoride (PVDF) 18
Positioning 37, 48, 51, 55, 57, 135, 137, 139
Postprocessing 41, 55, 196
Power 27, 29, 31, 65, 137, 192, 195, 196
  Output 27, 190
  Sonic 113
Pregnancy 78, 96
Preprocessing 41, 55, 196
Prosthesis 104
  Augmentation 104
  Breast 5
Pulse 22, 23, 42, 190, 195, 197
  Echo scanner 8
  Mechanical 18
  Short 24, 27, 38
  Ultrasound 22, 23, 42, 189, 190
  Voltage 18, 22, 24, 38
Radiation ix, 16
  Ionizing 90
  Therapy 131, 132
Radiography 7
  Specimen 8
Radiologist 6
Radiology viii
Range 196, 197
  Ambiguity 44
Receiver 15, 37, 38
Reflection 15, 18, 29, 32, 33, 44, 66, 133, 189, 190, 192-194, 196, 197, 199
Echogenic 67
Energy 15
Refraction 29, 32, 33, 41, 65, 66, 70, 71, 86, 87, 89, 92, 93, 97, 98, 118, 123, 137, 139, 191, 197
Region
  Anechoic 98, 189, 194
  Parenchymal 70, 76
  Retromammary 63, 70, 75, 78
  Subareolar 98
  Subcutaneous 63, 67, 70, 75, 78
Reid 3
Resolution 16, 19, 22, 23, 46, 51, 59, 190, 194, 195, 198, 199
  Axial 22, 24, 27, 59
  Cell 23
  Lateral 59, 60

Retromammary
  Fat (RMF) 75, 78, 96
  Region 63, 70, 75, 78
Reverberation 22, 197
  Artifact 16, 42, 43
Rib 65, 69, 75
Ring down 16
RMI breast phantom 58
Saline 104
Sarcoma 126
Scanner 19
  Ausonics dedicated breast 47
  Automated 33, 51
    Water path 51, 113
  Automatic breast 26, 51
  Breast ultrasound
    Dedicated 8
    Water path 3
  Pulse echo 8
  Ultrasound 3, 8
Scanning ix, 6, 18, 26, 41, 42-45, 48, 49, 51, 55, 57-59, 66, 89, 96, 137, 141, 195, 197-199
  Automated 5, 6, 8, 70, 135
  B-mode 23
  Static 42, 57
  Compound 41
  Contact 3, 15
  Hand-held 6, 23, 32, 41, 135
  Real-time 5, 8, 23, 32, 41, 42, 48, 193
  Tank 53
  Transducer 51
  Water path 32, 66
Scar 99, 135
Scattering 15, 16, 18, 25, 26, 189, 190, 192, 197, 199
Sclerosing adenosis 135, 136
Screen, intensifying 17
Segmentectomy 131
Selenium-coated aluminum plate 17
Septation 98
Septum 46, 63, 89
Shadowing 26, 27, 33, 43, 66, 67, 70, 71, 75, 87, 89, 92, 93, 98, 106, 109, 111-113, 117, 120, 121, 123, 125, 131, 132, 135-137, 140, 196
Silicone 103-106
Skin 15, 16, 21, 25, 37, 42, 50, 55, 63, 65-67, 70, 73, 75, 94, 99, 109, 111, 113, 114, 119, 121, 131, 132, 135, 137, 197
Slice, 48, 51, 57, 193, 197
  Diagonal 57
  Longitudinal 57
  Sagittal 53
  Thickness 46, 53, 59, 60, 195, 198
  Transverse 53, 57
Slider 38, 55
Sonography vii-ix, 3-5, 15, 37, 48, 50, 51, 57, 59, 63, 70,

75, 83, 95, 97-99, 109, 111, 116, 117, 120, 122, 124-126
  Automated 4, 7, 37
  Breast x, 3
  False-positive 135
  Imaging 113, 117
  Transmission computerized 7
Sonomammography 4, 66, 109, 133, 135
Sound 15, 24, 26
  Beam 57, 99
  Intensity 27
  Power 113
  Transmission 32
  Wave 8, 15-17, 26, 29, 37, 40, 49, 70, 71, 199
Spectrum 25
  Frequency 24
Spiculation 117, 134
Sponge 42, 43, 59
Stain
  Eosin 110, 116
  Hematoxylin 110, 116
Storage assignment 41
Stroma 90, 92, 110
Subcutaneous
  Fat 28, 29
    Globule 69
  Region 63, 67, 70, 75
Surgery 99, 118, 131, 132
Tank 55, 137
  Scanning 53
  Water 51, 53, 59, 139
  Bath 140
Technicare (unit) 53, 59, 72, 76, 86, 94, 96, 112, 119, 121, 132, 134, 141
Technique ix, x, 35-61
Technologist x, 4, 27, 37, 38, 51, 53, 55, 57, 141, 191
Tendon 25
Testis 25
Texture 40, 41, 99, 189, 194, 197, 198
Therapy 5
  Radiation 131, 132
Thorax 63
Thread 44-46, 53, 59, 60, 199
Time gain compensation (TGC) 26, 27, 29, 30, 37, 38, 43, 53, 55, 57, 59, 60, 140, 189, 196, 198, 199
Tissue 7, 8, 15, 16, 19, 22-27, 29, 32, 33, 41, 42, 46, 63, 65, 67, 78, 88, 89, 92, 102, 135, 137, 190, 192-199
  Brain 25
  Breast vii, viii, 8, 15, 16, 24, 25, 37, 38, 59, 95, 104, 111, 117, 135, 137, 196
  Cell 192, 197
  Compliance 6
  Connective 63, 65-67, 70, 75, 90-92, 95, 109, 113, 117, 120, 135

204 breast ultrasound

Fatty 98, 111, 123, 135
Fibroglandular 84
Glandular 25, 29, 75, 137
Heart 25
Hyperechoic 40
Kidney 25
Liver 25
Parenchymal 7, 26, 65, 67, 70, 72, 75, 111, 133, 135
Penetration 16
Subareolar 98
Subcutaneous 16
Tendon 25
Testis 25
Toner
   Powdered 17
Transducer 5, 6, 8, 15-19, 21-27, 32, 33, 37, 38, 40-44, 47-57, 60, 74, 114, 133, 137, 141, 189-199
   Array 190
      Annular 8
   Ausonics 59
   Automated 32
   Beam 137
   Element center 47
   Frequency 190
   Hand-held 19, 23, 32, 37, 49
   Higher frequency viii, 6, 8, 16, 27, 198
   Mechanically moving 42
   Motor-driven 23, 24
   Multidirectional 66
   Real-time 19, 23, 51, 98
      Scanning 51
   Technicare 59
   Ultrasound 16
   Wafer 19
Transmission
   A-mode 189
   Computerized sonography 7
   Energy 15
   Ultrasound 189
Trauma 189
Traumatic hemorrhage 131
Trigger level 55
Tumor 32, 38, 90, 92, 109-111, 113, 117, 120, 123
   Benign 26, 90, 91

Breast 8
   Epithelial 95, 111
   Malignant 26, 122
   Solid 28, 29, 46, 90
Ultrasonic
   Computerized axial tomography (UCAT) 7, 8
   Scanner 8
   Speckle 8
Ultrasound vii, ix, x, 3-6, 15-17, 25-27, 33, 37, 38, 41, 49, 63, 65, 70, 72, 83, 87, 90, 95, 103, 104, 109, 113, 114, 117, 120, 121, 131-133, 136, 189, 190, 192, 194, 195, 197-199
   Abdominal viii
   Absorption 25
   Amplitude 191
   Automated 86, 96, 134, 141
   Baseline 48
   Beam 33, 65, 67, 70, 75, 111, 133, 190, 191, 196, 197
   Breast vii, viii, 3-8, 15, 28, 37, 73, 131, 133, 136
      Automated vii, 4, 7
      Hand-held vii
   Dedicated 8, 77, 86, 88, 93, 112, 119
   Echo 44
   Energy 70, 113
      Wave 15
   Examination 6, 37, 70, 104, 106, 131, 132
   False-negative 134
   Frequency 25
   Hand-held 84, 97, 101, 114, 123
   Imaging vii-ix, 7, 8, 15, 16, 18, 25, 28, 29, 37, 40, 49, 63, 75, 95, 113, 133, 197, 198
   Impedance 29
   Lens 195
   Mammography vii, 4, 16, 75, 104, 137
   Obstetrical viii
   Parenchymal 70
   Phantom

Breast 59
Pulse 22, 23, 42, 189, 190
Real-time 37, 84, 97, 101, 114, 141
Scanner 3, 8
Transducer 16
Unit 196, 199
Wafer 18
Wave 15, 18, 25, 26, 29, 32, 33, 38, 41, 190, 192-196, 198, 199
Unit 42, 44, 53, 57, 141, 192
   Array 46
   Ausonics 53, 54, 59, 141
   Automated 41, 42, 46
      Breast scanning 51
      Scanning 70
   B-mode 56
   Hand-held 41
   Labsonics 56, 59
   Mechanical 42-44, 46
   Phased 46
   Philips 38
   Real-time 41, 42, 193, 196
      Electrical 42
      Mechanical 42
   Technicare 53, 59, 141
   Ultrasound 196, 199

Vessel 133
Videodisc 6
Videotape 37
   Dual 6
Voltage 15, 17-19, 24, 27, 40, 189, 192-196, 198
   Pulse 22, 24, 38

Wafer 18, 19, 22-24, 195
   Ceramic 195
   Piezoelectric 18, 24, 33, 189, 190, 195, 199
   Transducer 19
   Ultrasound 18
Water 19, 42, 43, 58, 59, 66, 113, 189, 194
   Bag 43, 53, 57, 58, 189
   Offset 23, 32, 33
   Spacer 141
   Bath 52, 53, 56, 197
      Polyethylene-enclosed 57

Tank 140
Delay mechanism viii
Gap 19
Offset 23, 32, 33, 43, 46, 47
Path 15, 139
   Automated 6, 19
   Breast ultrasound scanner 3
   Examination 137
   Scan 32, 66
   Step-off device 6, 97
   Tank 51, 53, 59, 139
Water-soluble acoustic gel 17
Wave 15, 16, 18, 19, 22-24, 32, 33, 37, 40, 191, 193-198
   Energy 15
   Frequency 24, 25
      High 15, 24, 25
      Low 25
   Mechanical 15, 16, 18, 27, 189, 195
   Moire 41, 195
   Sound 8, 15-17, 26, 29, 37, 40, 49, 70, 71, 199
   Ultrasound 15, 18, 25, 26, 29, 32, 33, 38, 41, 190, 192-196, 198, 199
Wavelength 47, 192, 194, 195, 199
Wild 3
Windowing 41
Wolfe 70

Xeromammography 4, 17, 122
Xeroradiography 18
X-ray viii, 4, 16, 18, 37, 75, 90, 131
   Abnormality 131
   Examination 90, 104
   Focal spot 16
   Imaging 16
   Mammography vii-ix, 4-8, 15-18, 37, 63, 70, 71, 75, 90, 104, 106, 109, 111, 113, 117, 120, 133, 135, 136, 141
   Photon 17
   Tube 16